MOUNTAIN WARRIORS

by Anna Kekesi-Kim

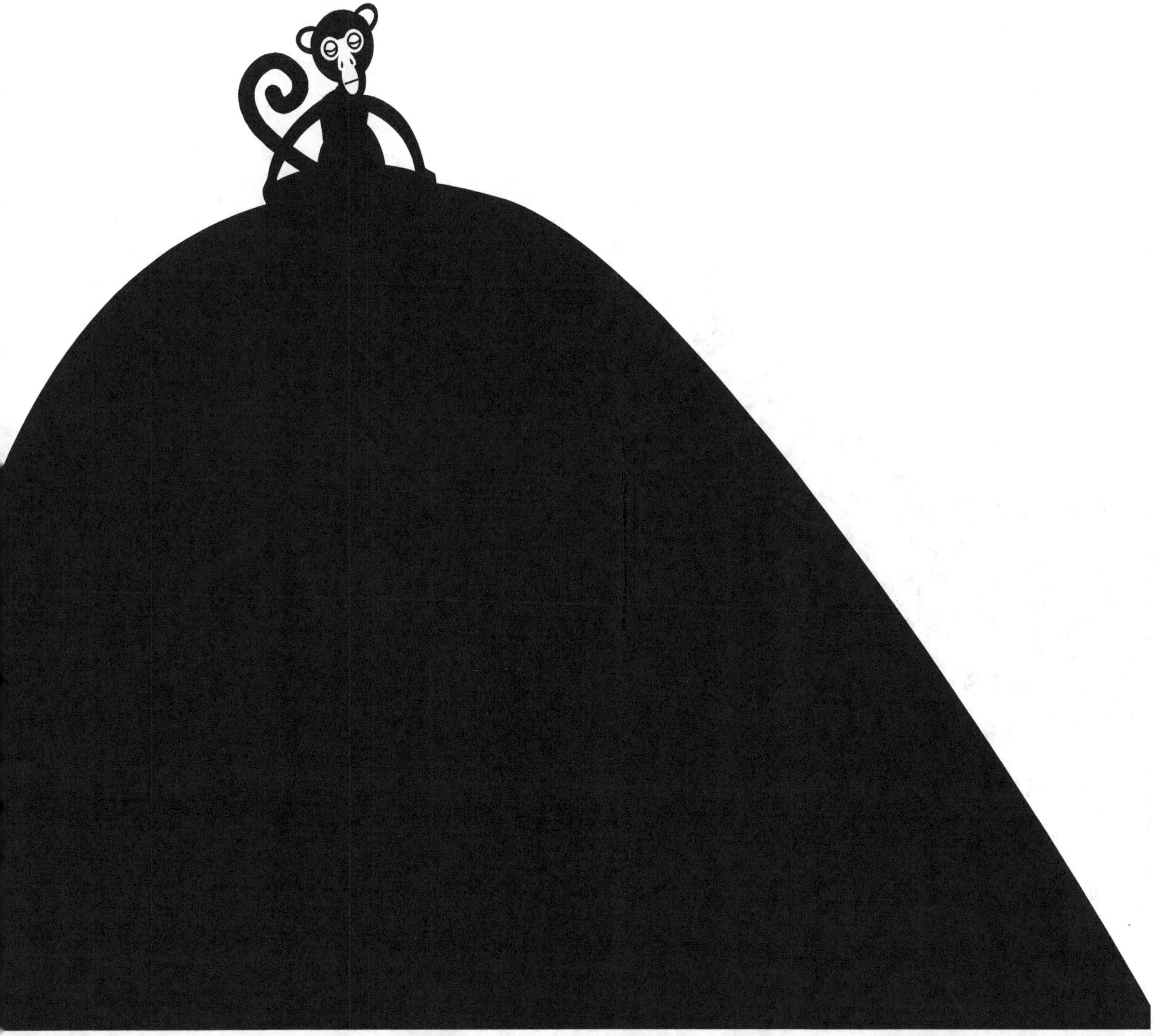

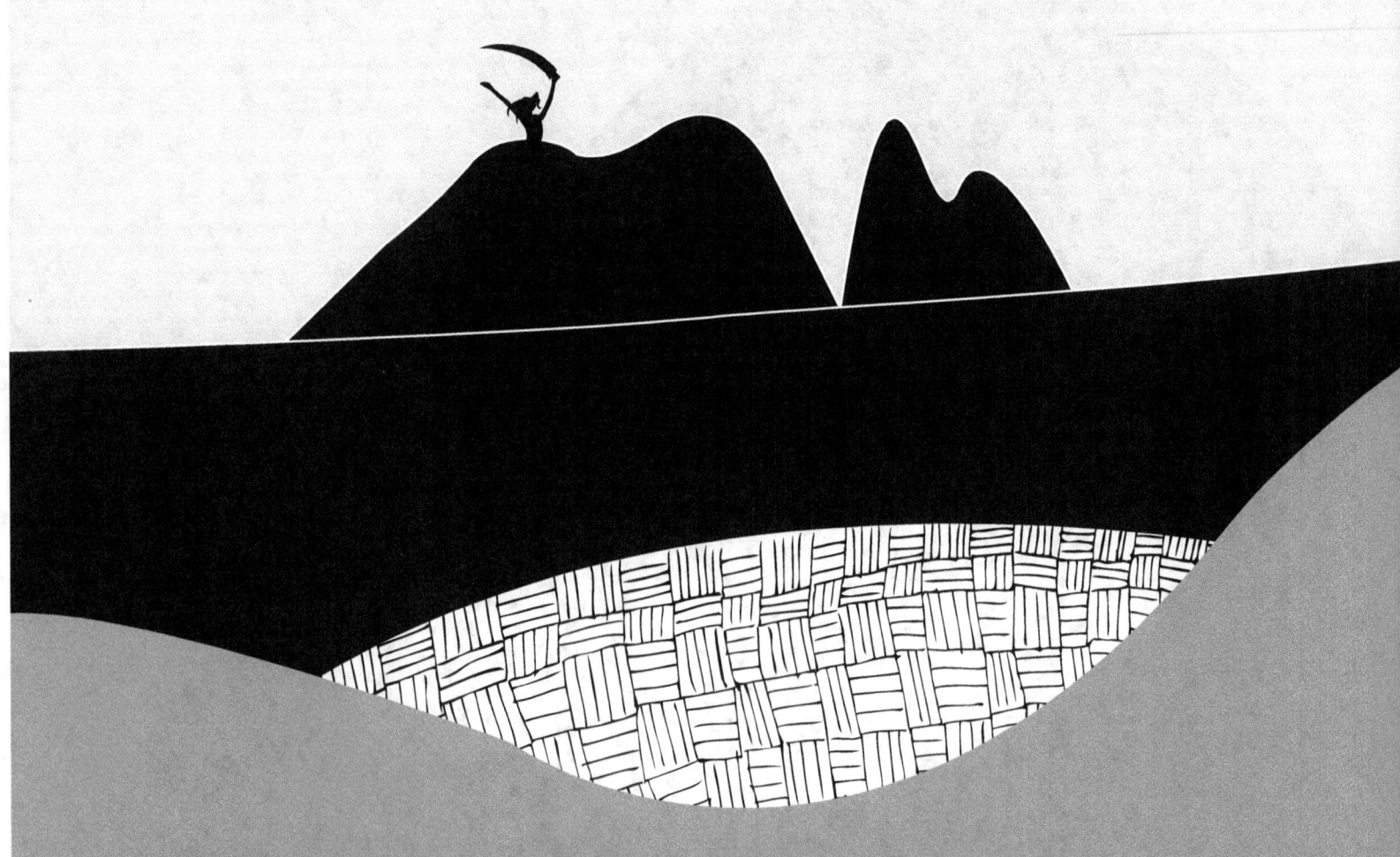

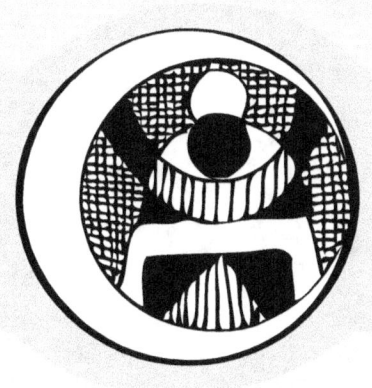

for my Monkey

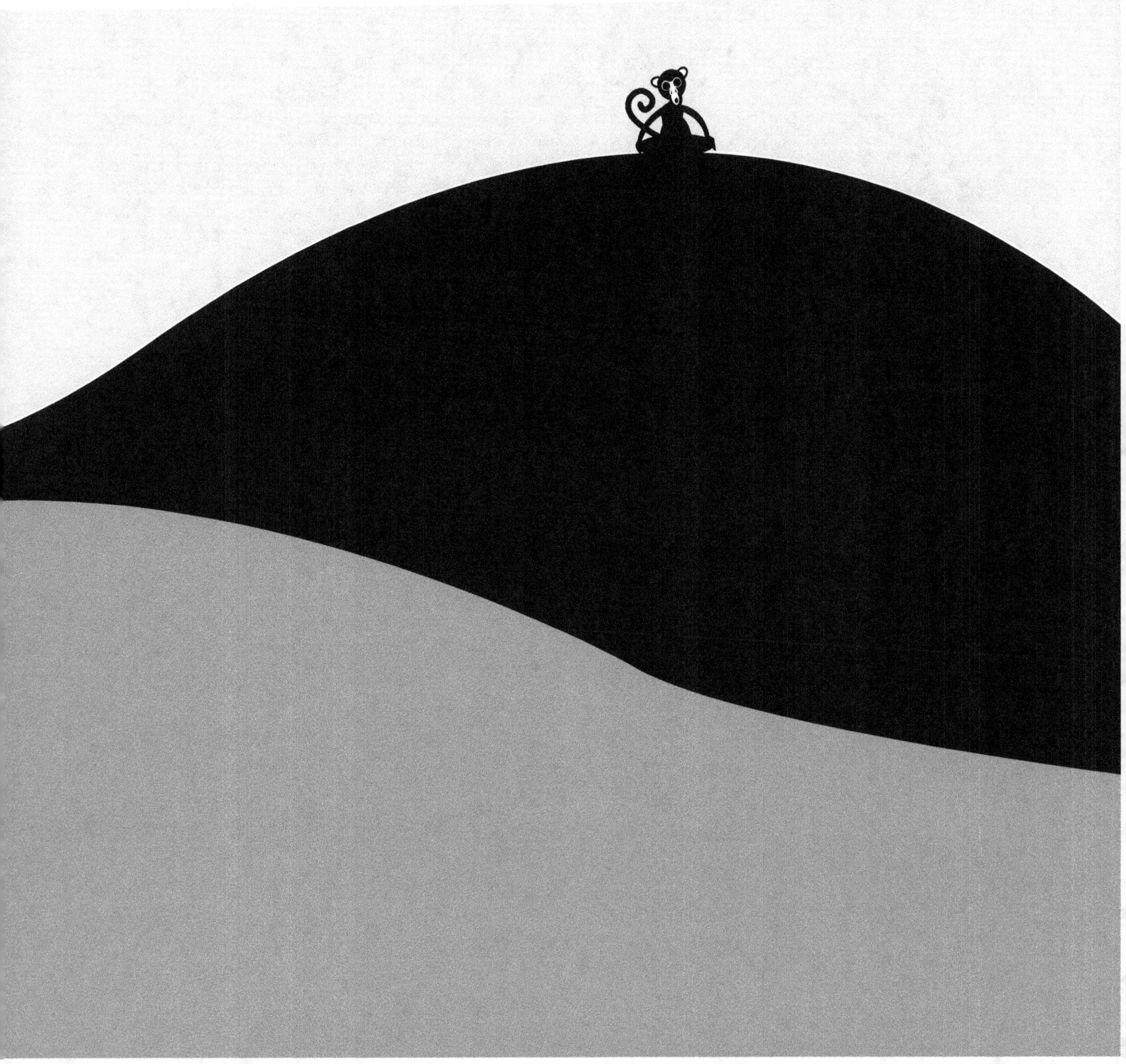

AUTHOR'S NOTE:

Yoga is a way for young children to explore their bodies and quiet their minds. Please remember to use caution when introducing any physical activity. In this story, only a few yoga poses are introduced. Remind the children to listen to their bodies and never do any poses that hurt. This book is not intended to replace proper yoga teacher training. Only practice poses that you are already familiar with. Encourage the children to be the characters that they meet in the story and to make some noise. Breathe, relax and enjoy.

Namaste

Mountain was sleeping.
so he didn't know…

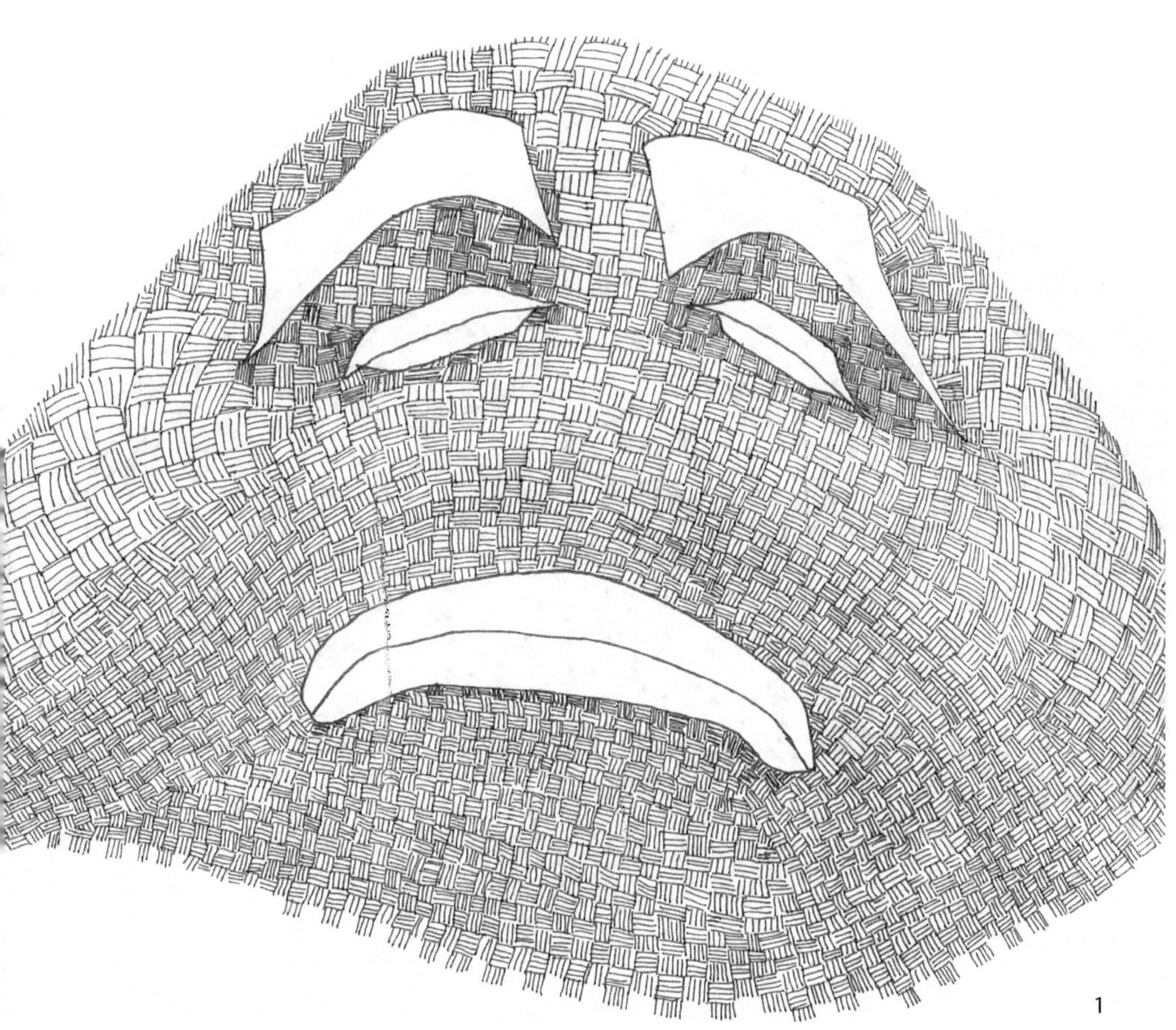

That the warriors were coming.

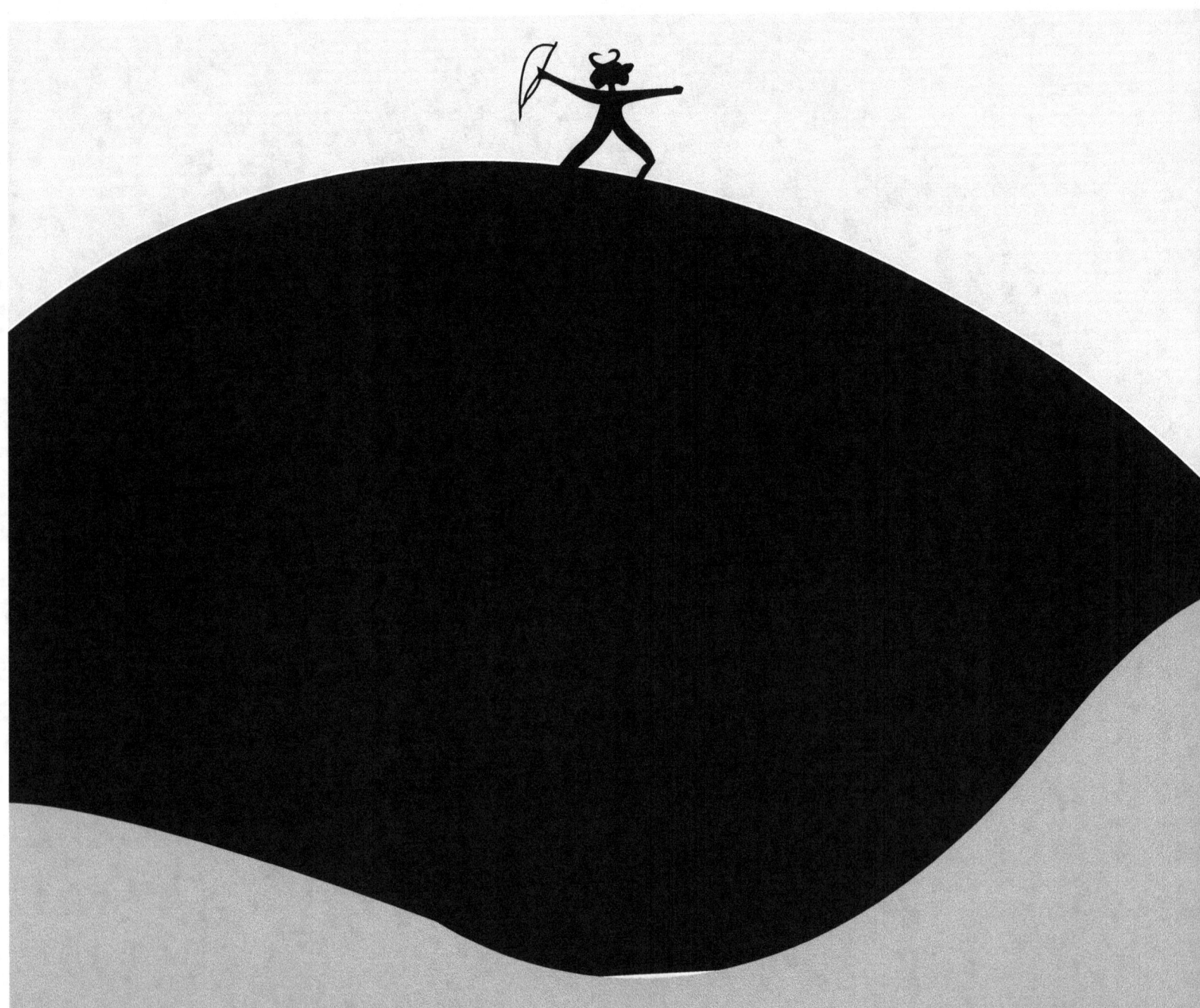

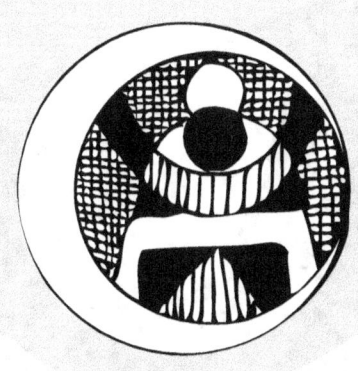

Santosha Swan saw the warriors coming.

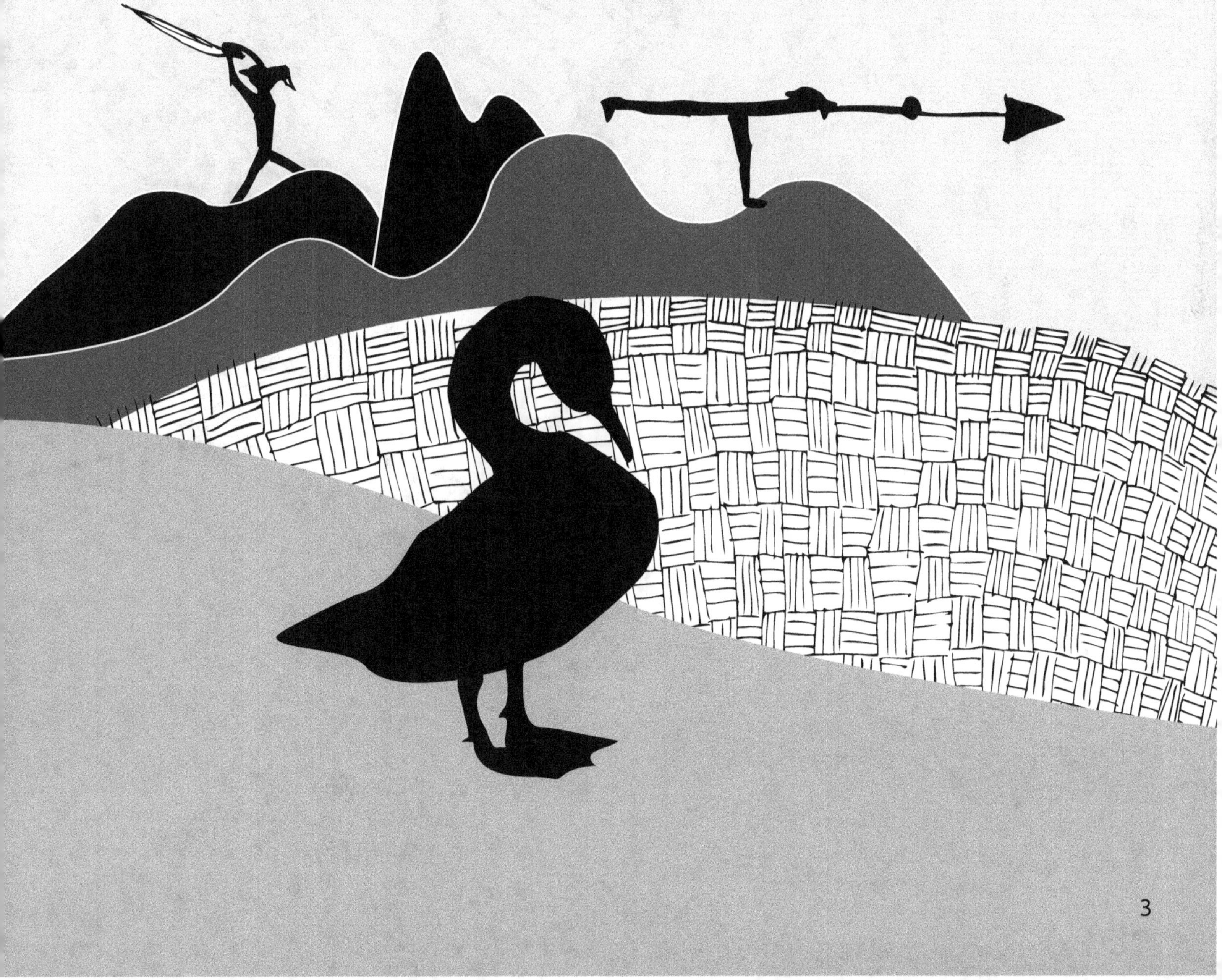

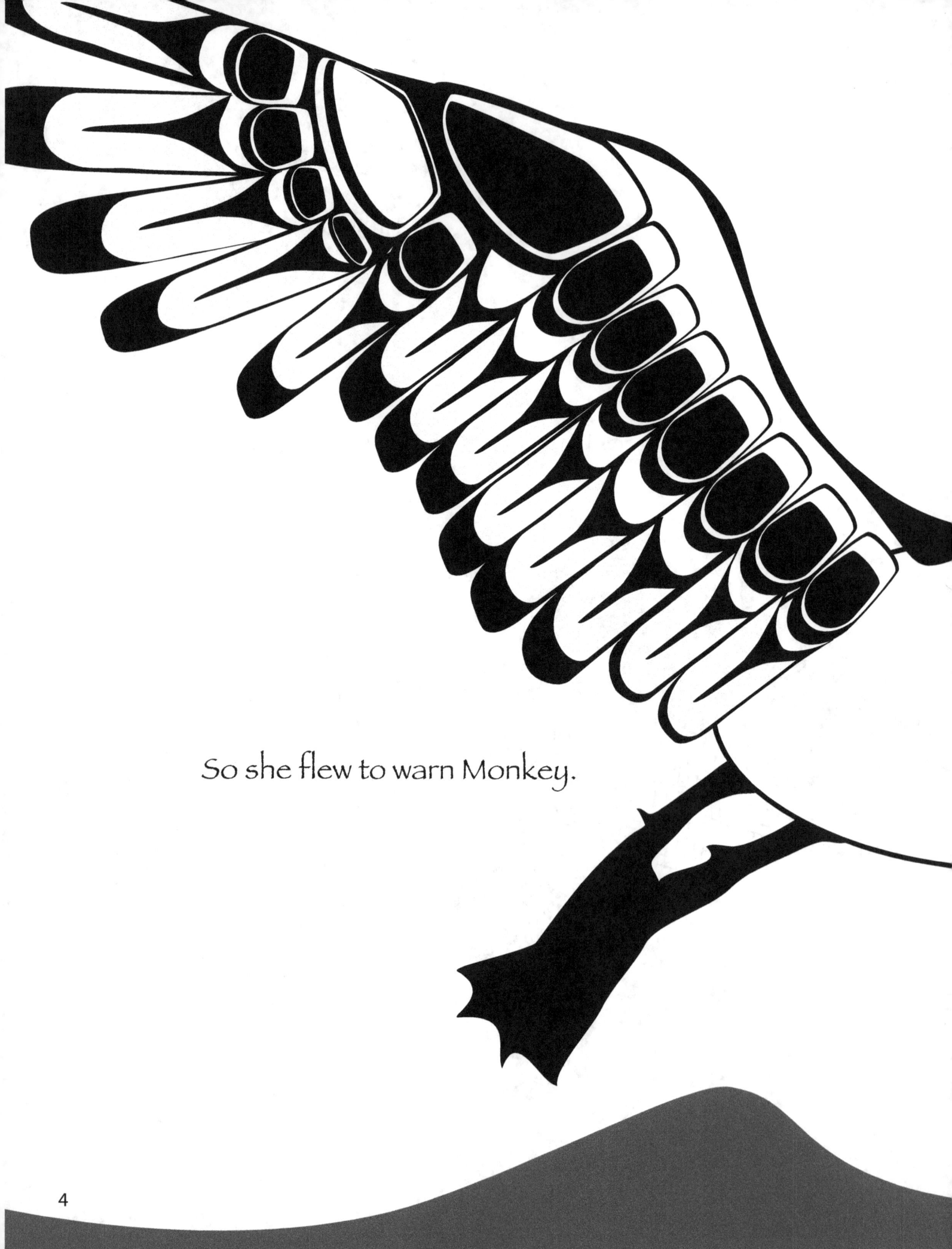

So she flew to warn Monkey.

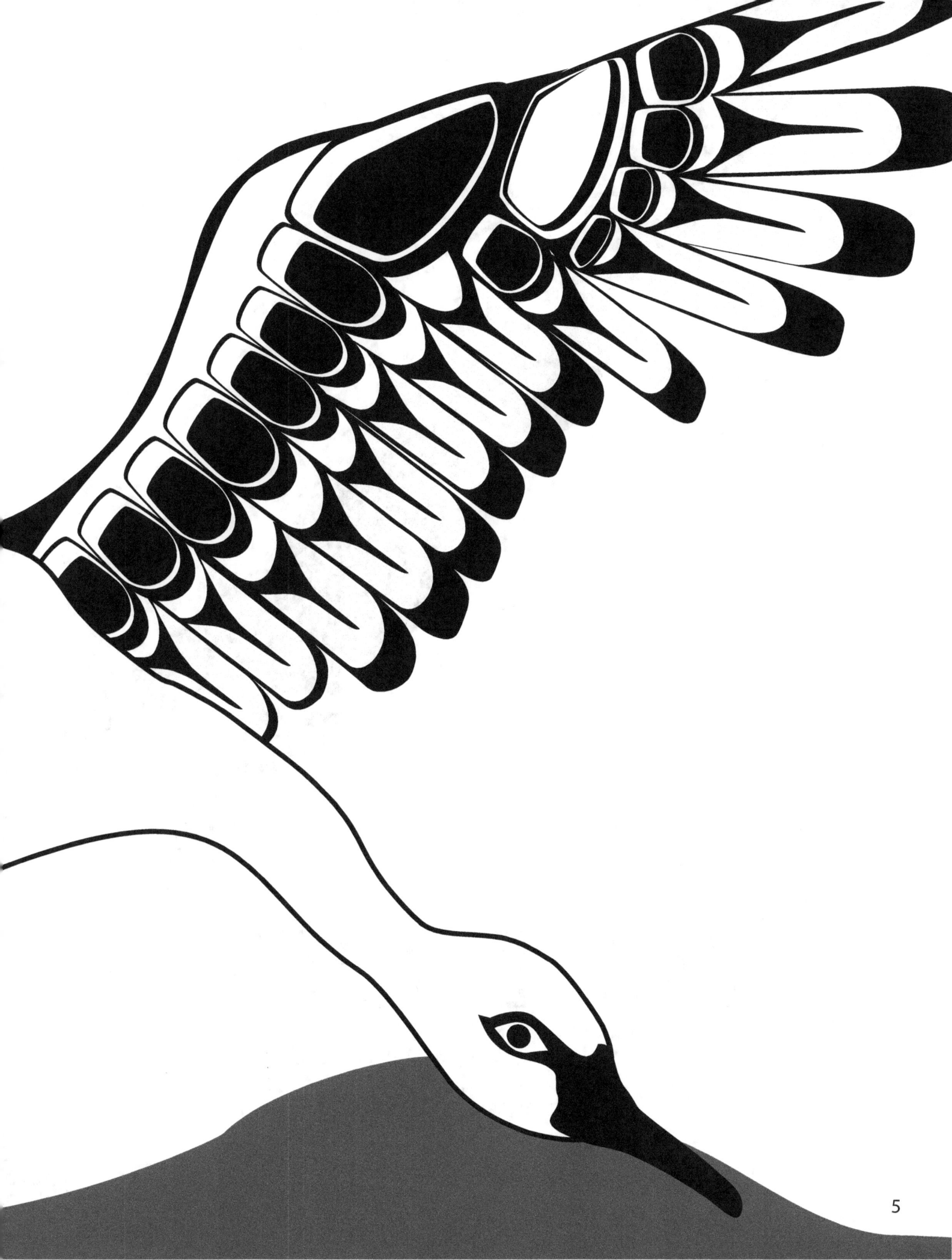

5

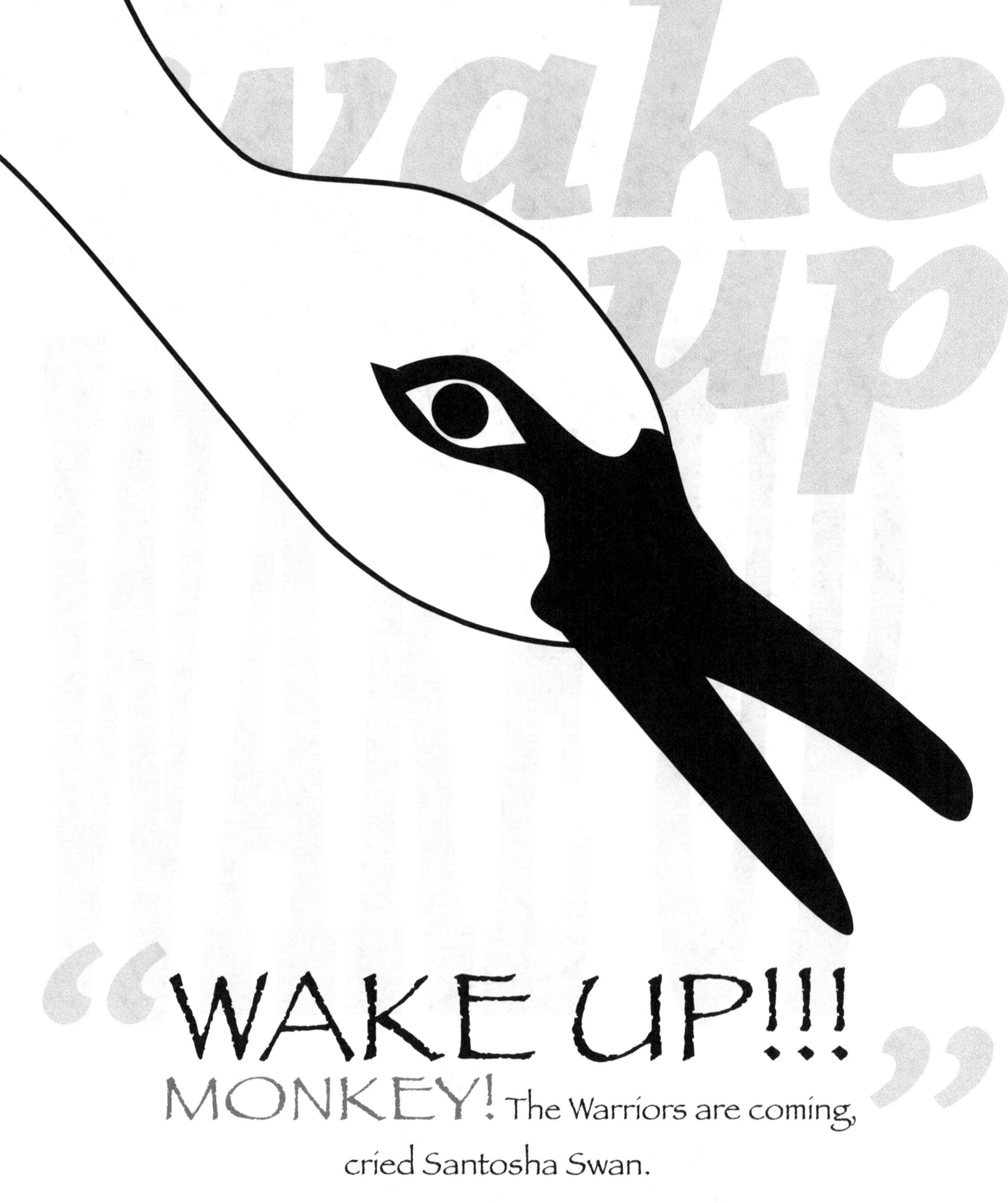

"**WAKE UP!!!**
MONKEY! The Warriors are coming, cried Santosha Swan.

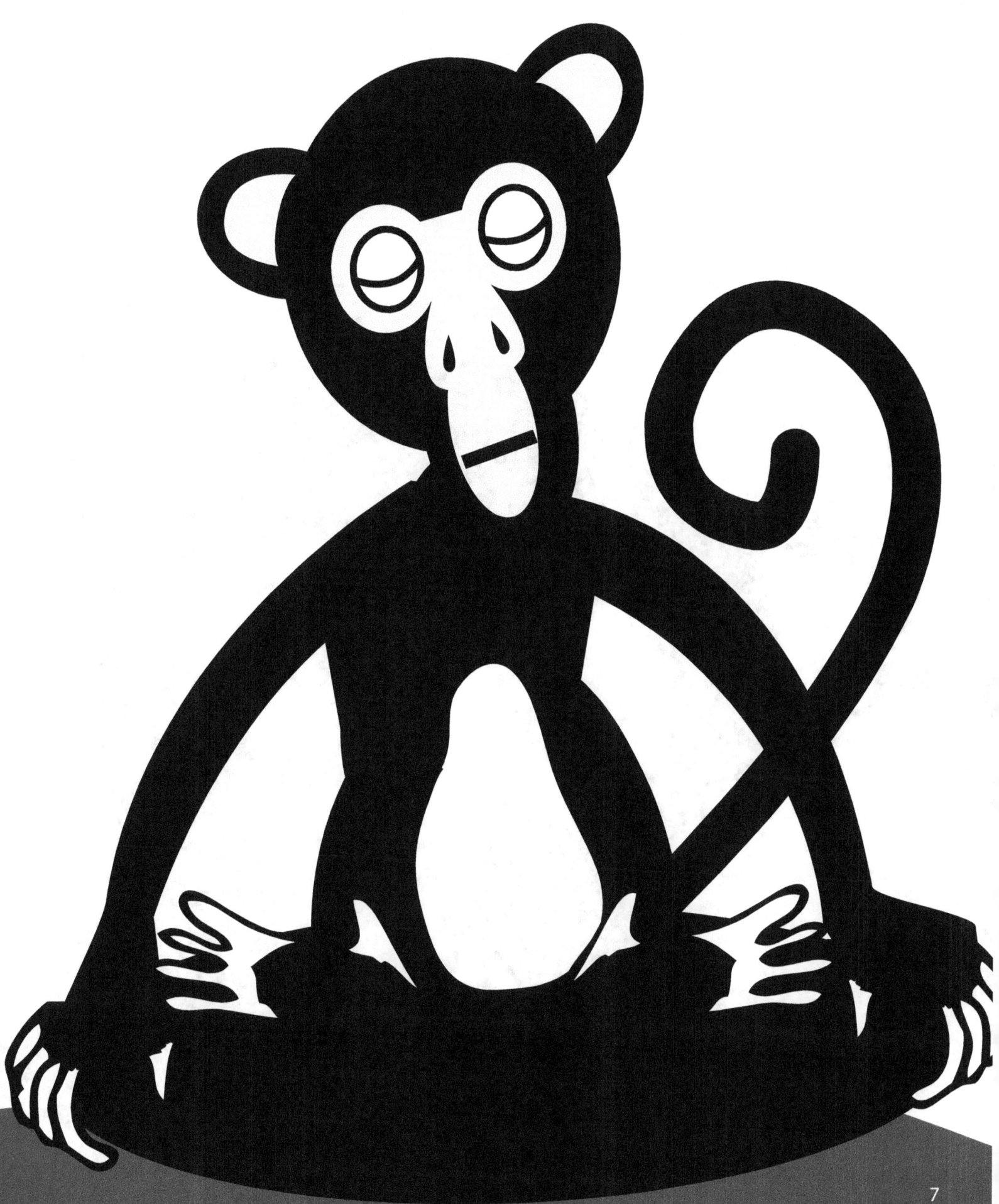

OOOOOOO

OOOOOO

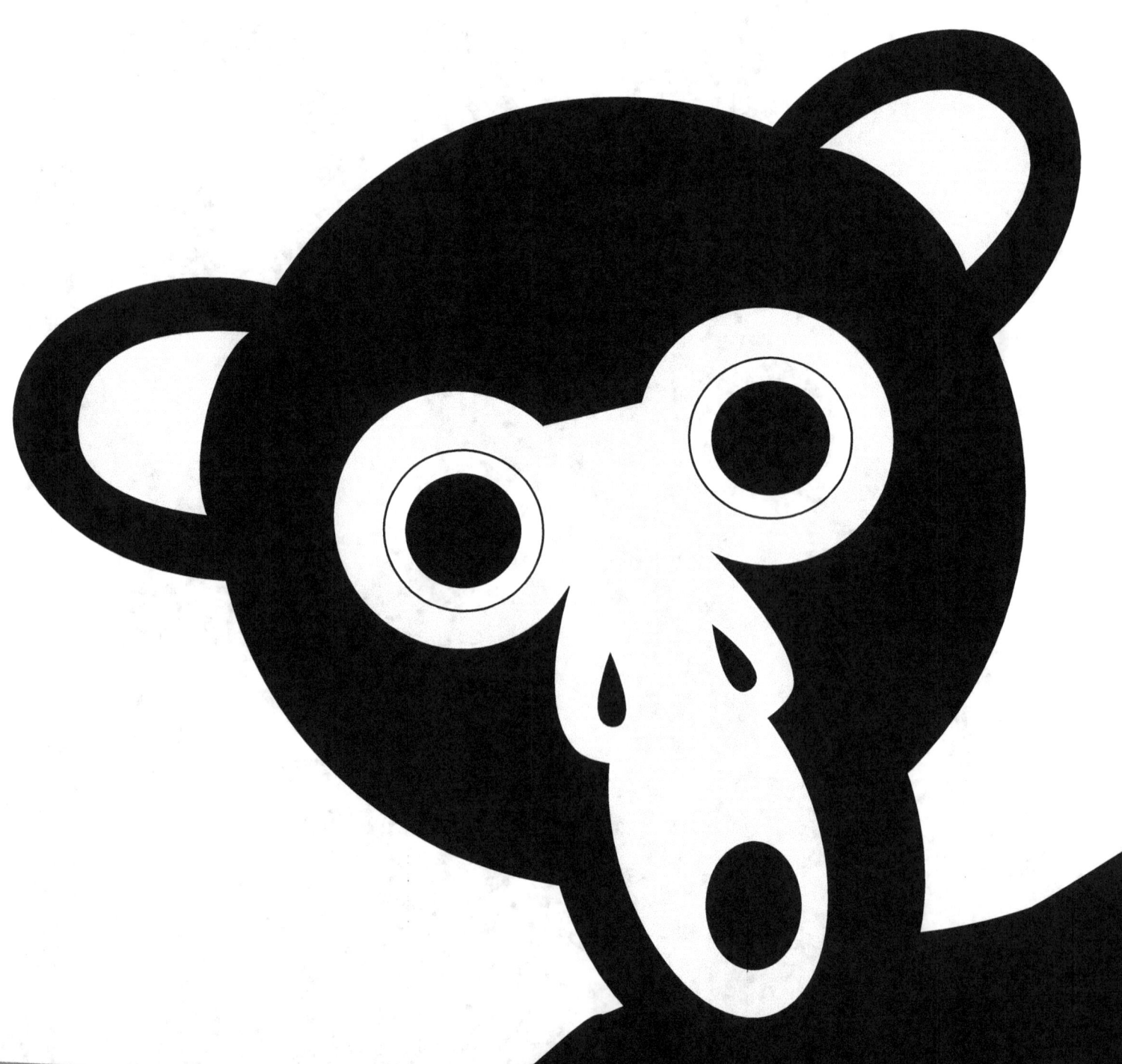

"**OOOO OOOOO**"

moaned Monkey.

"I know," said Santosha Swan, "we have to warn everyone that the Warriors are coming."

SWOOSH

OOOOO

SWOOSH

They raced to Mountain.
Santosha Swan swooped,
diving to the ground.
Monkey followed,
reaching forward.

First Santosha Swan,
then Monkey,
then Swan ,
then Monkey again.

swoosh *oooo*

SWOOSH SWOOSH SWOOSH

O O O O O

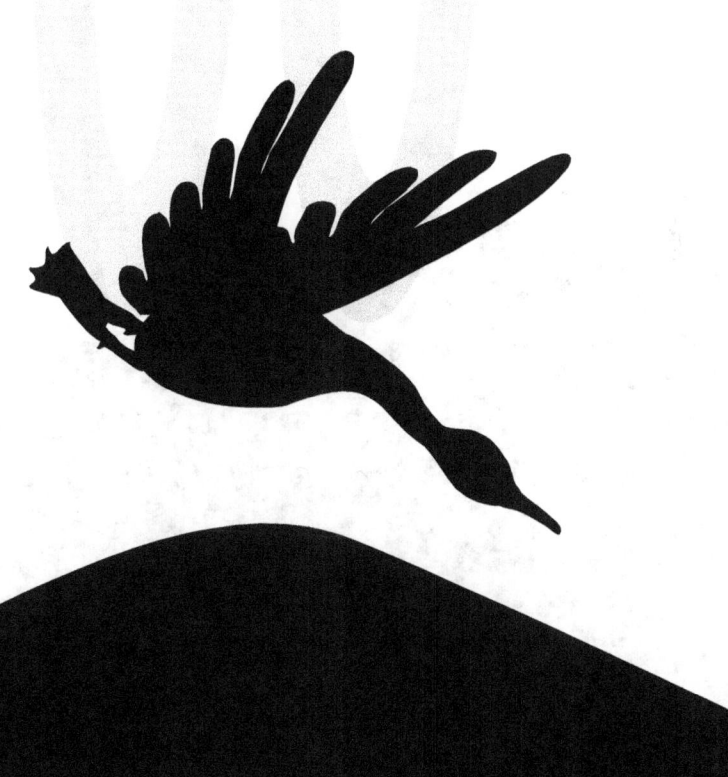

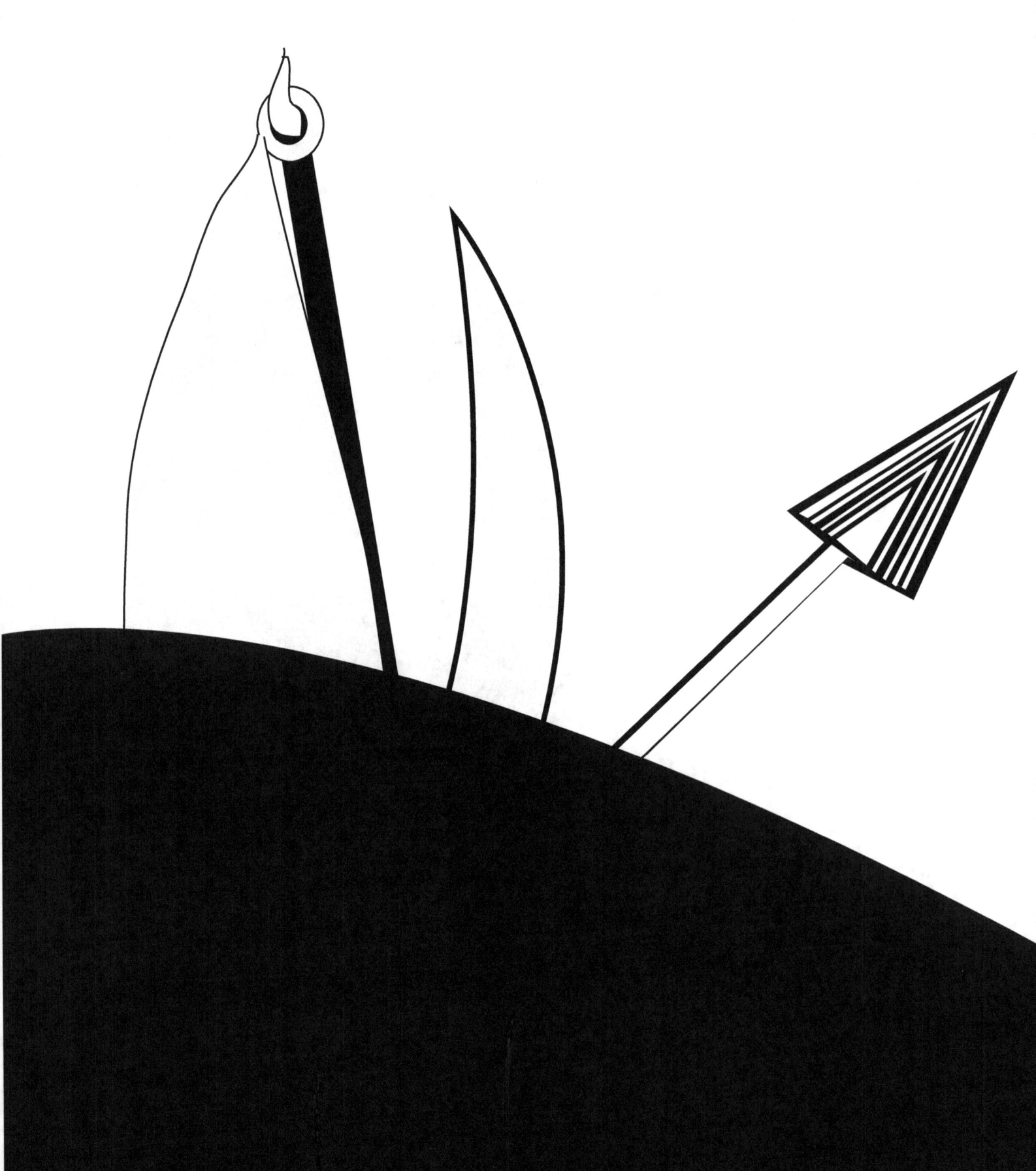

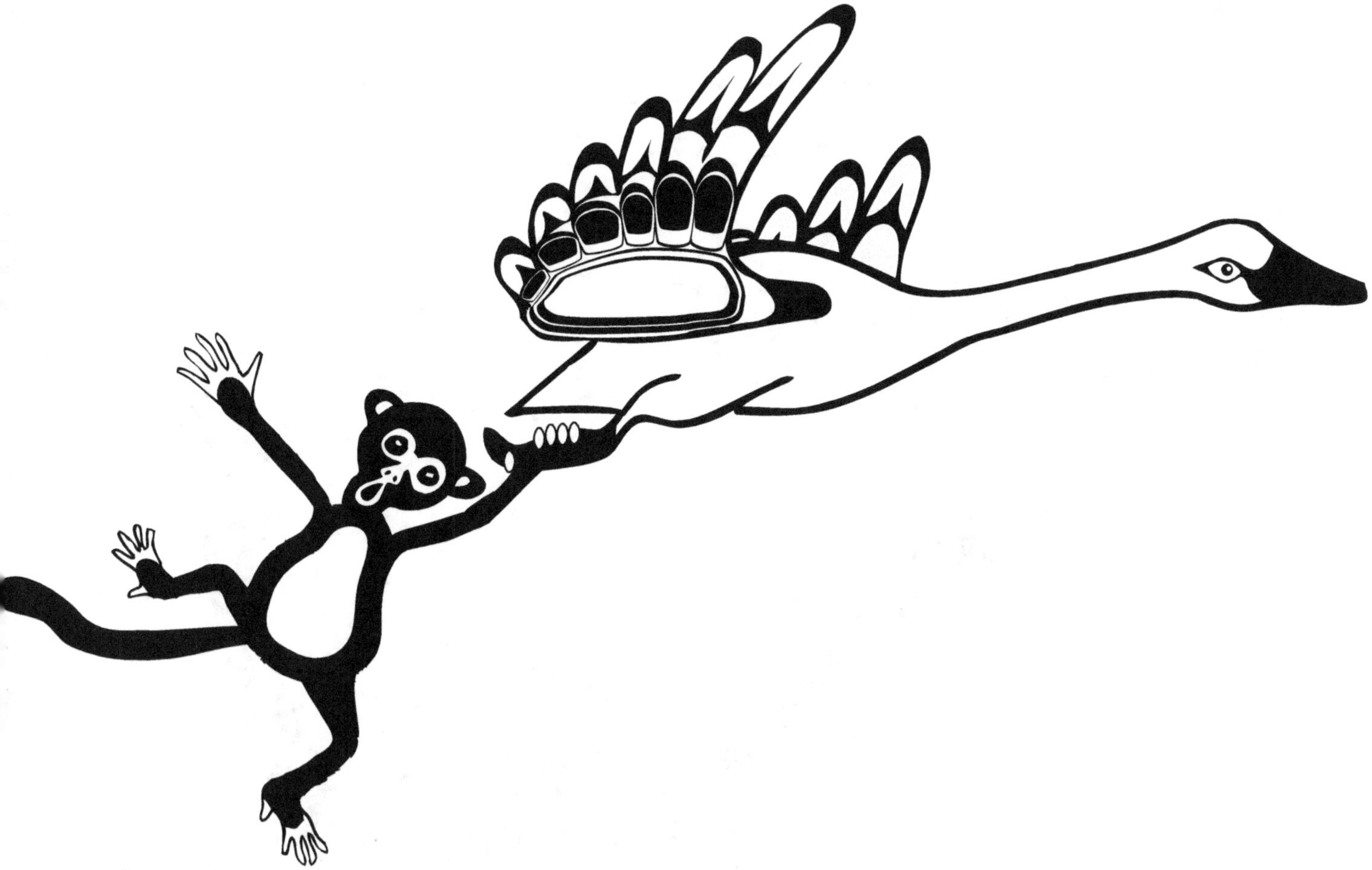

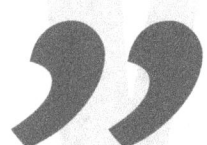

"HURRY,

THEY ARE GETTING CLOSER!!"

trumpeted Swan.

Warrior 1 stood tall and proud.
He hummed,

"*LAAM*

LAAM."

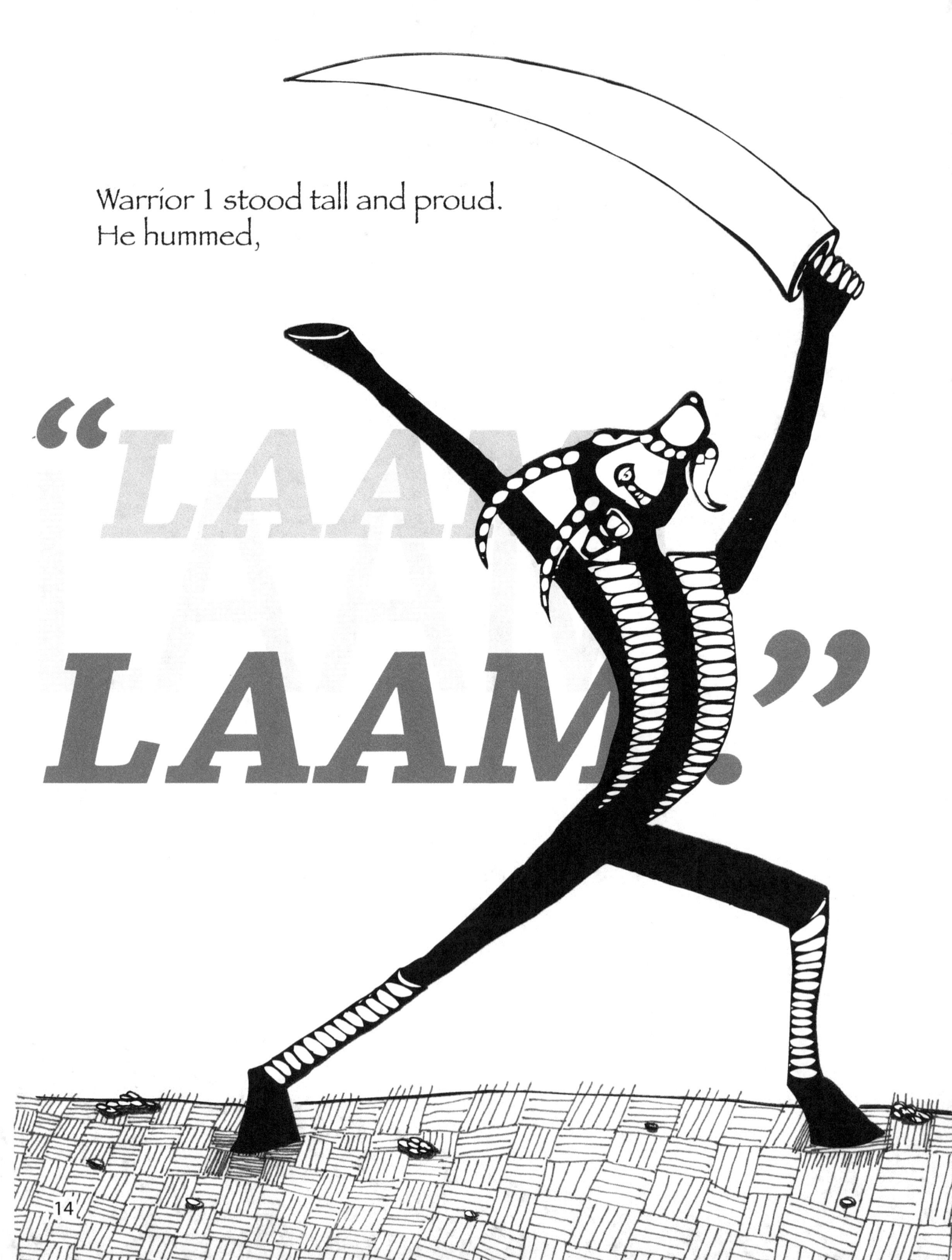

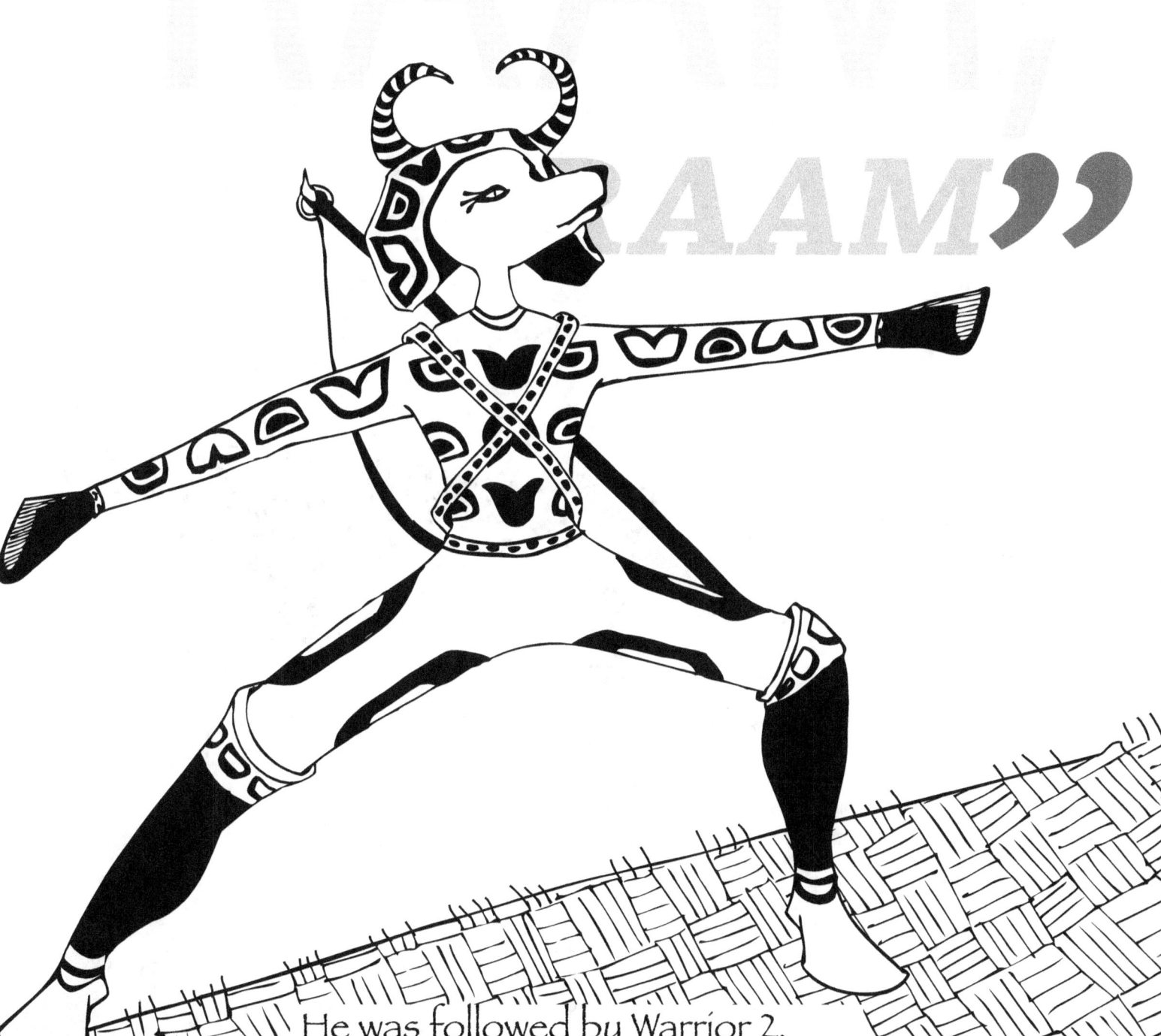

"RAAM, RAAM, RAAM"

He was followed by Warrior 2. She was strong and reached long as she sung her own song,

15

Warrior 3 followed, balancing on one leg as she chanted,

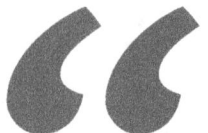 *VAAM,*

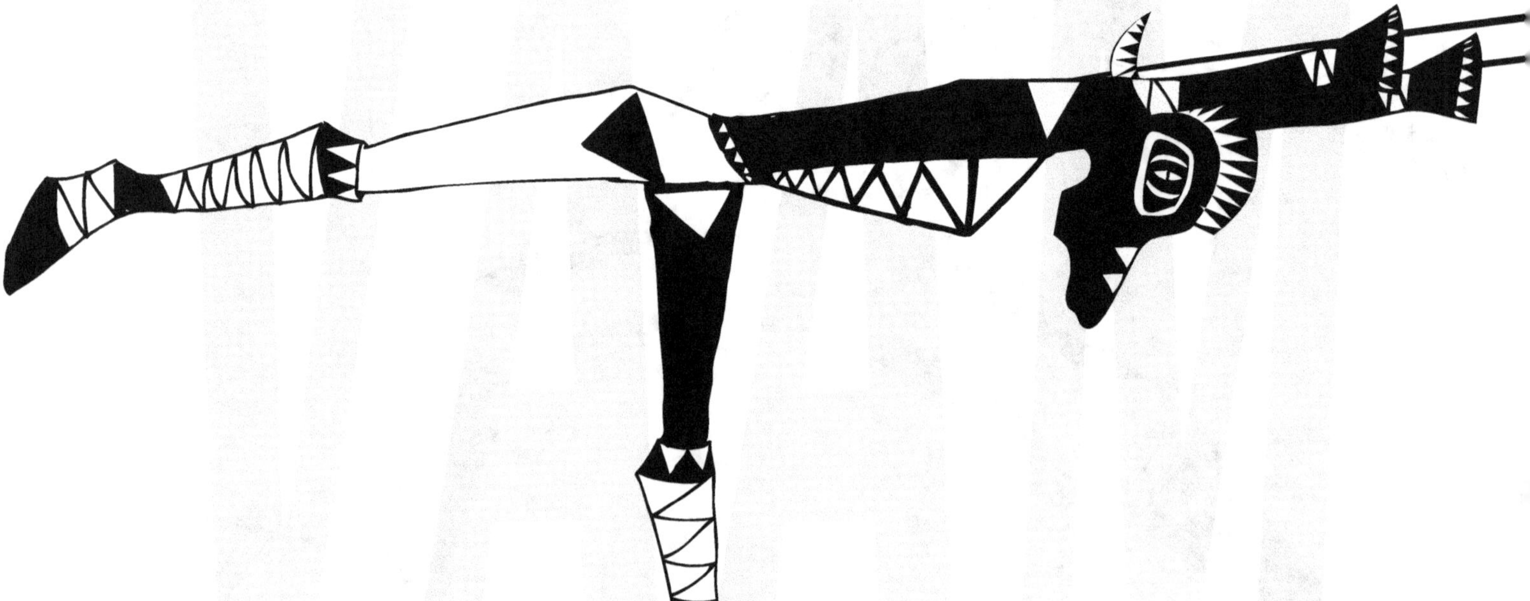

VAAM.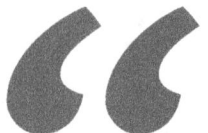

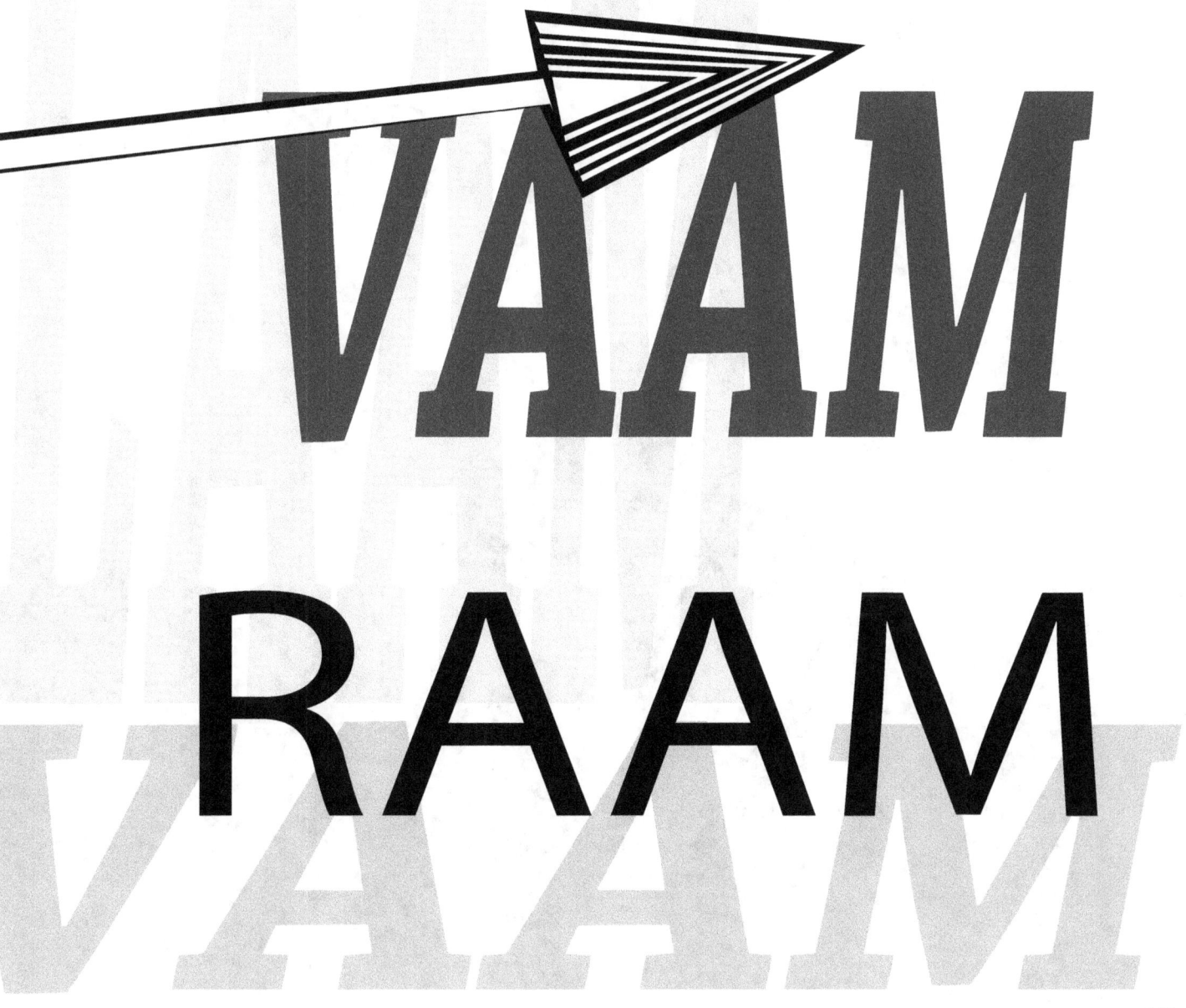

LAAM.

RAAM.

VAAM

RAAM

17

LAAM
VAAM
RAAM

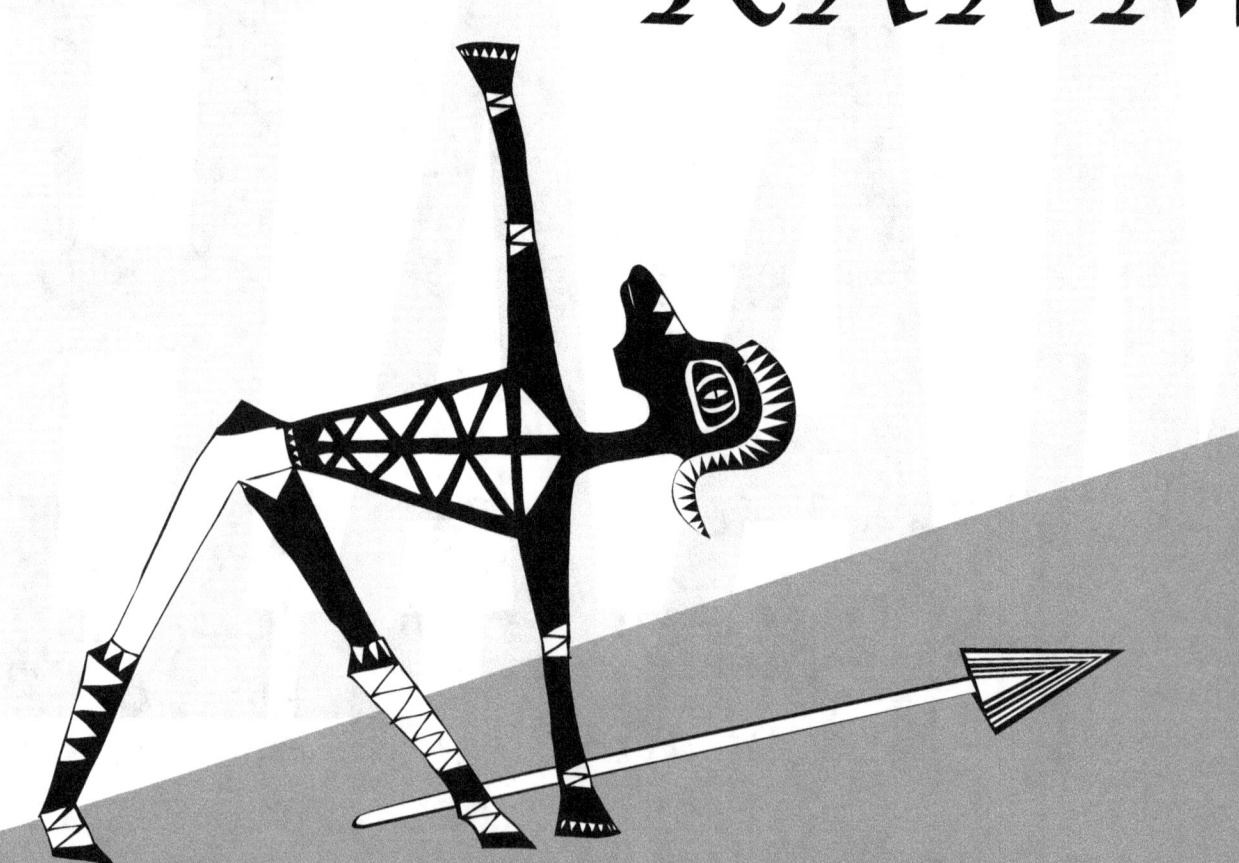

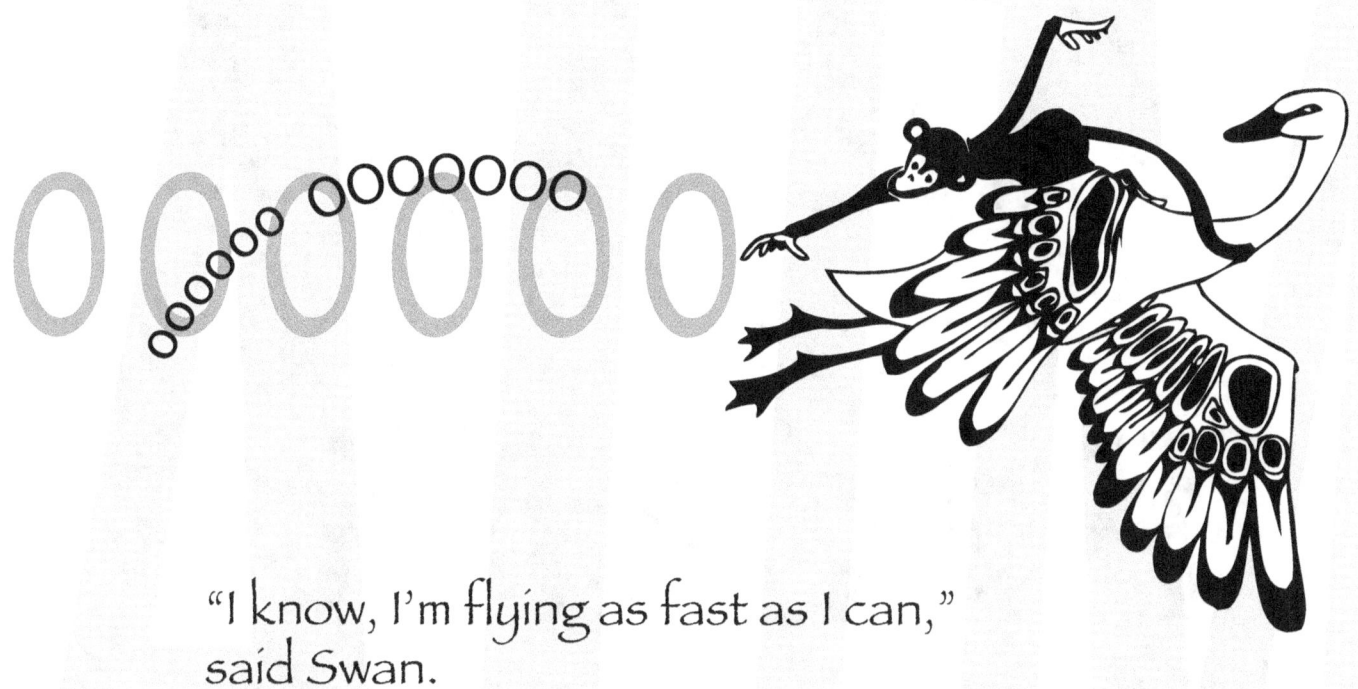

"I know, I'm flying as fast as I can,"
said Swan.

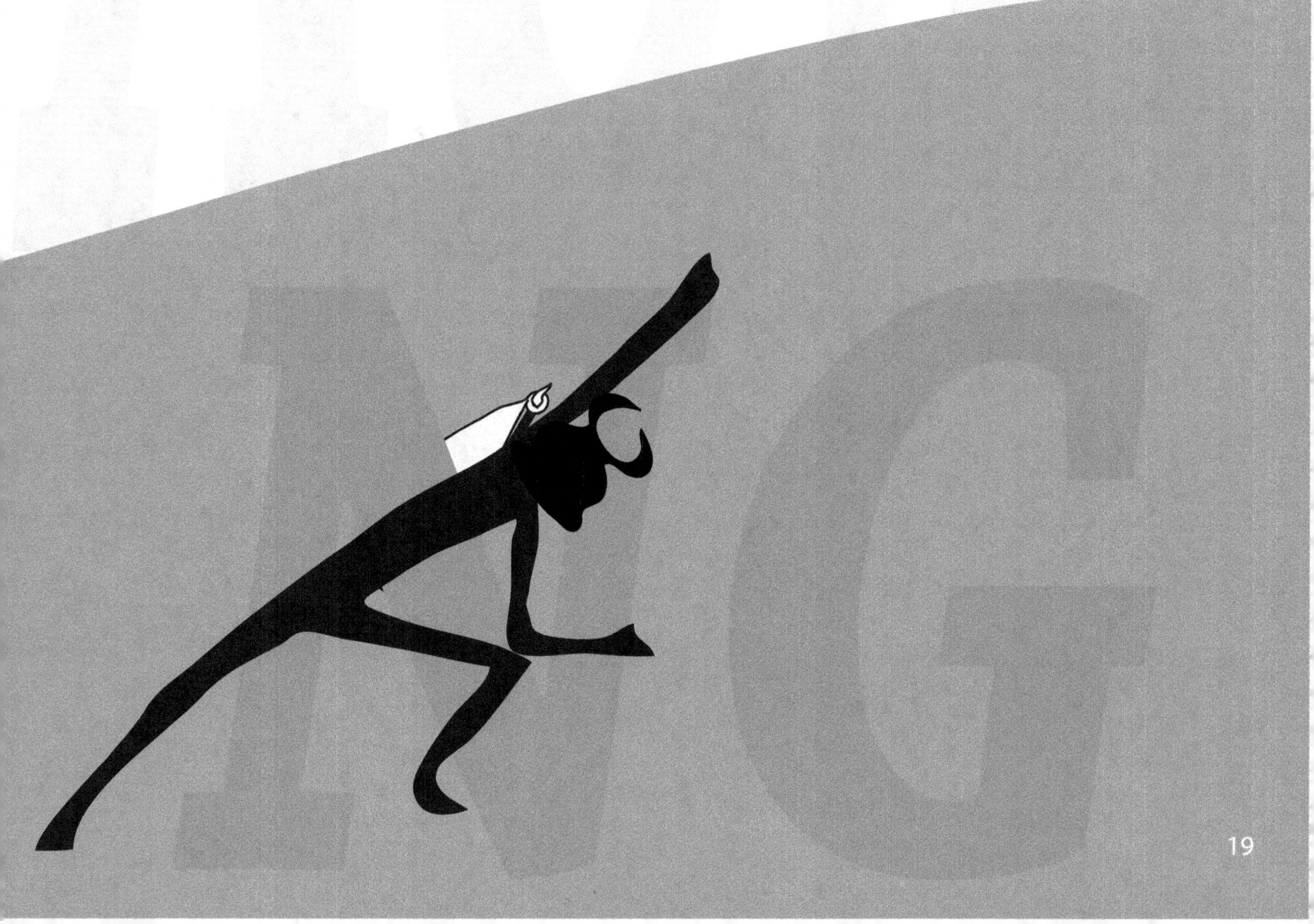

LAAM

VAAM

RAAM

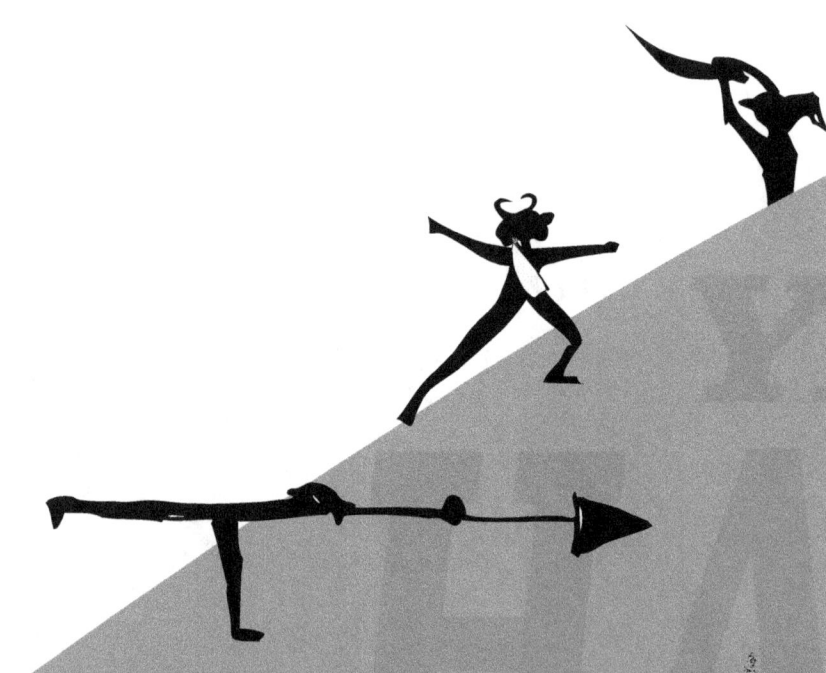

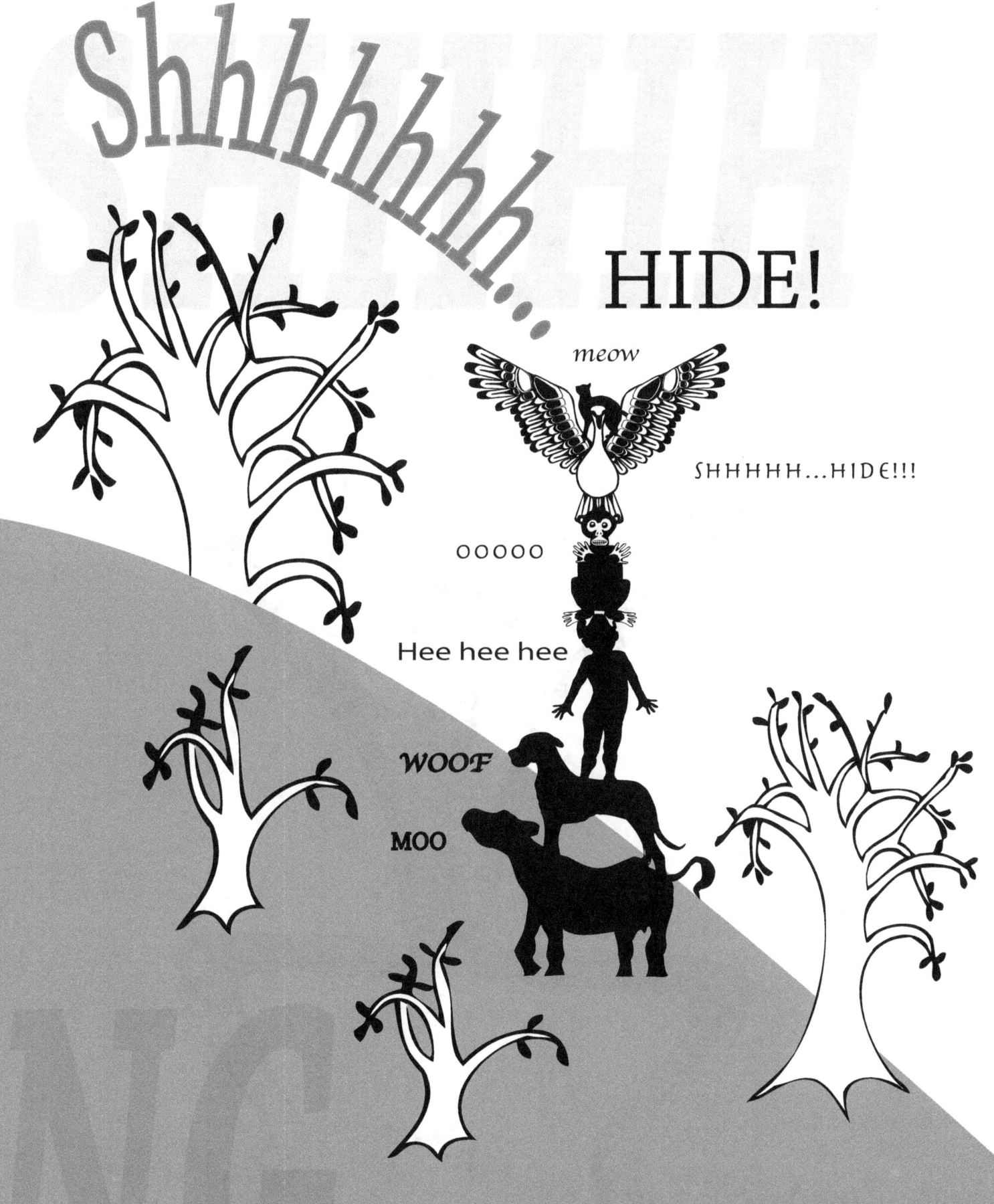

"Where did they go?" wondered Warrior 1.

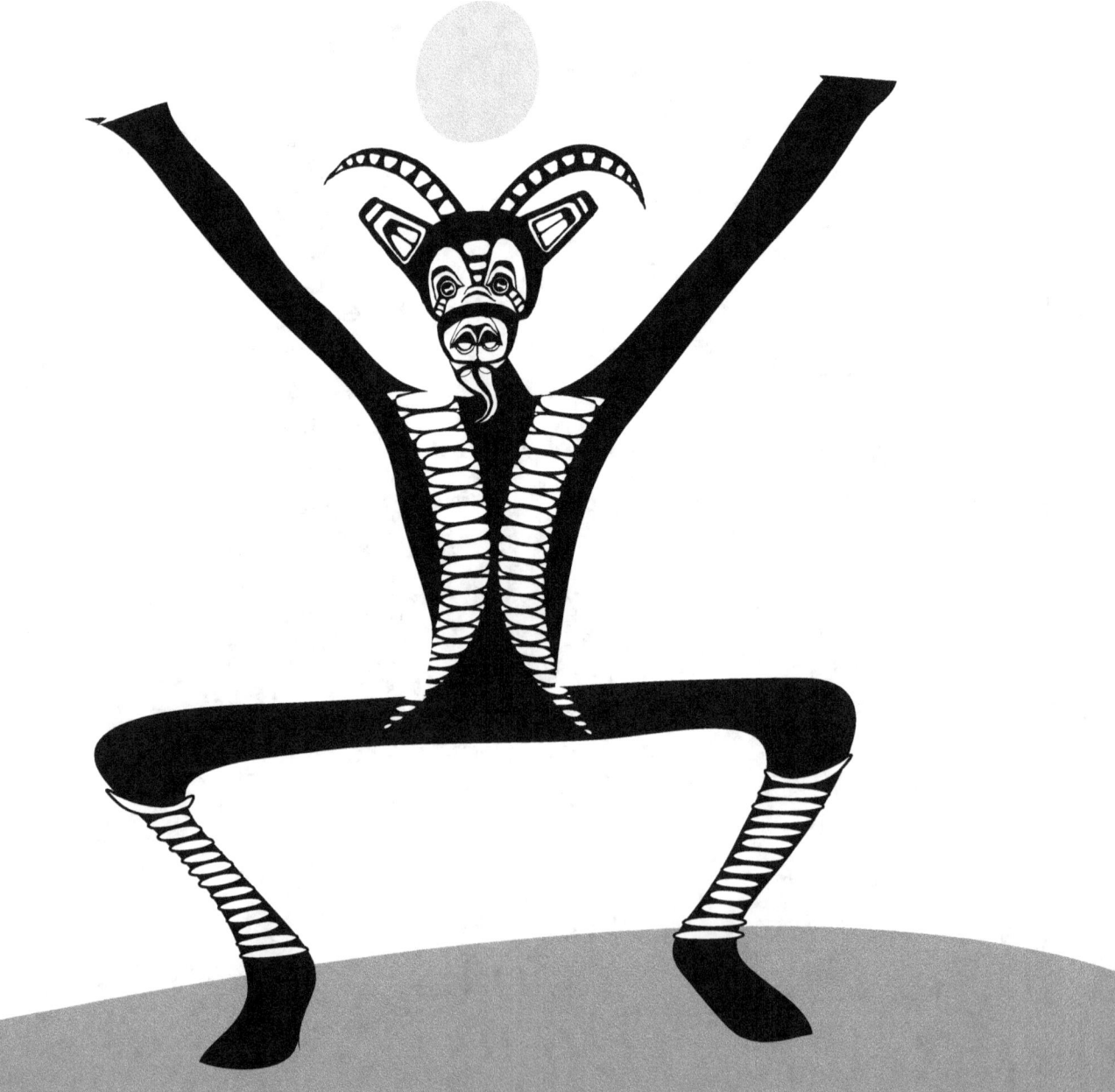

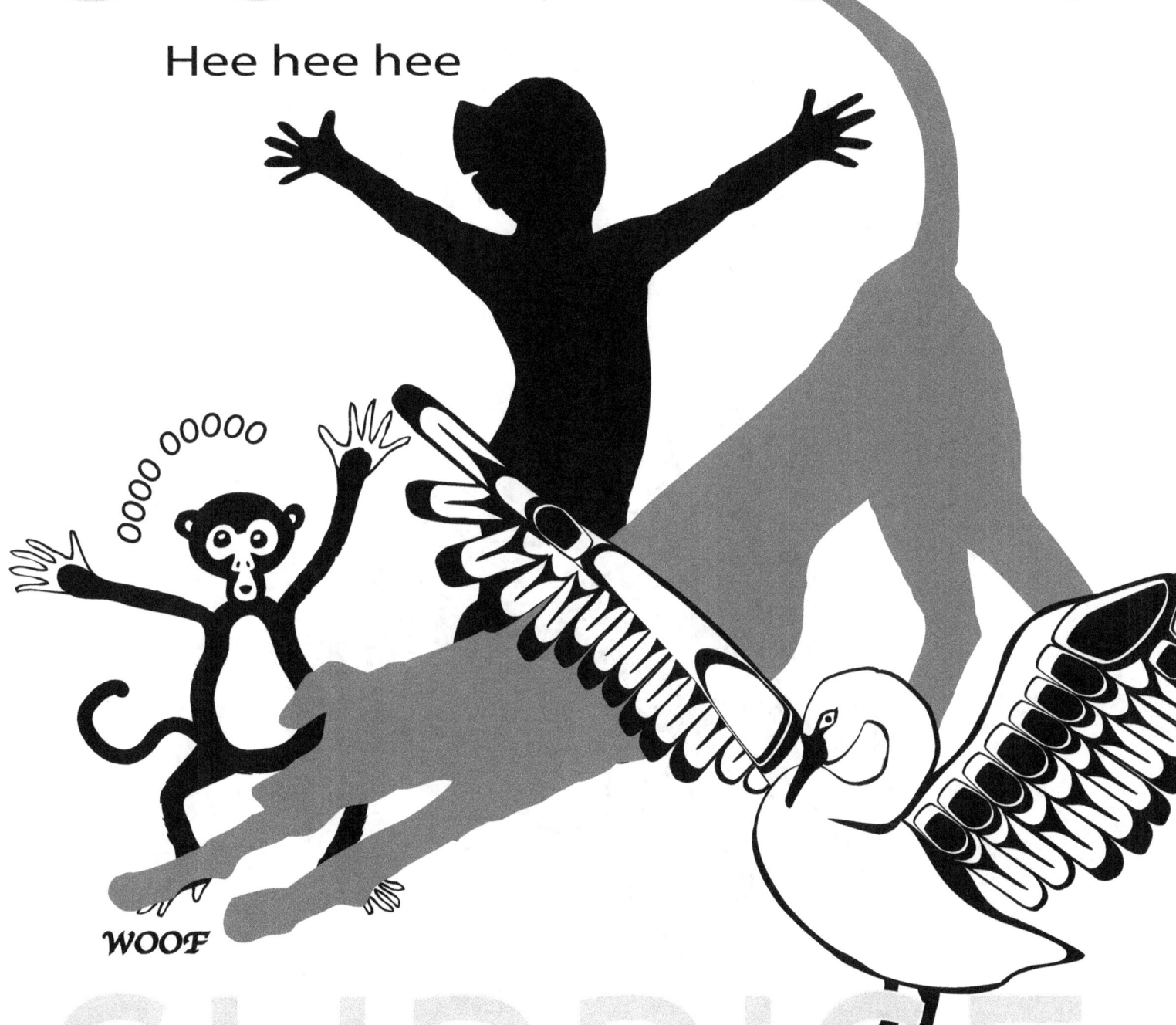

23

"Are we too late?" cried Swan.
"Santosha, you made it just in time," said Warrior 2.
"How can we help?" asked Swan.
"You can help us unpack."

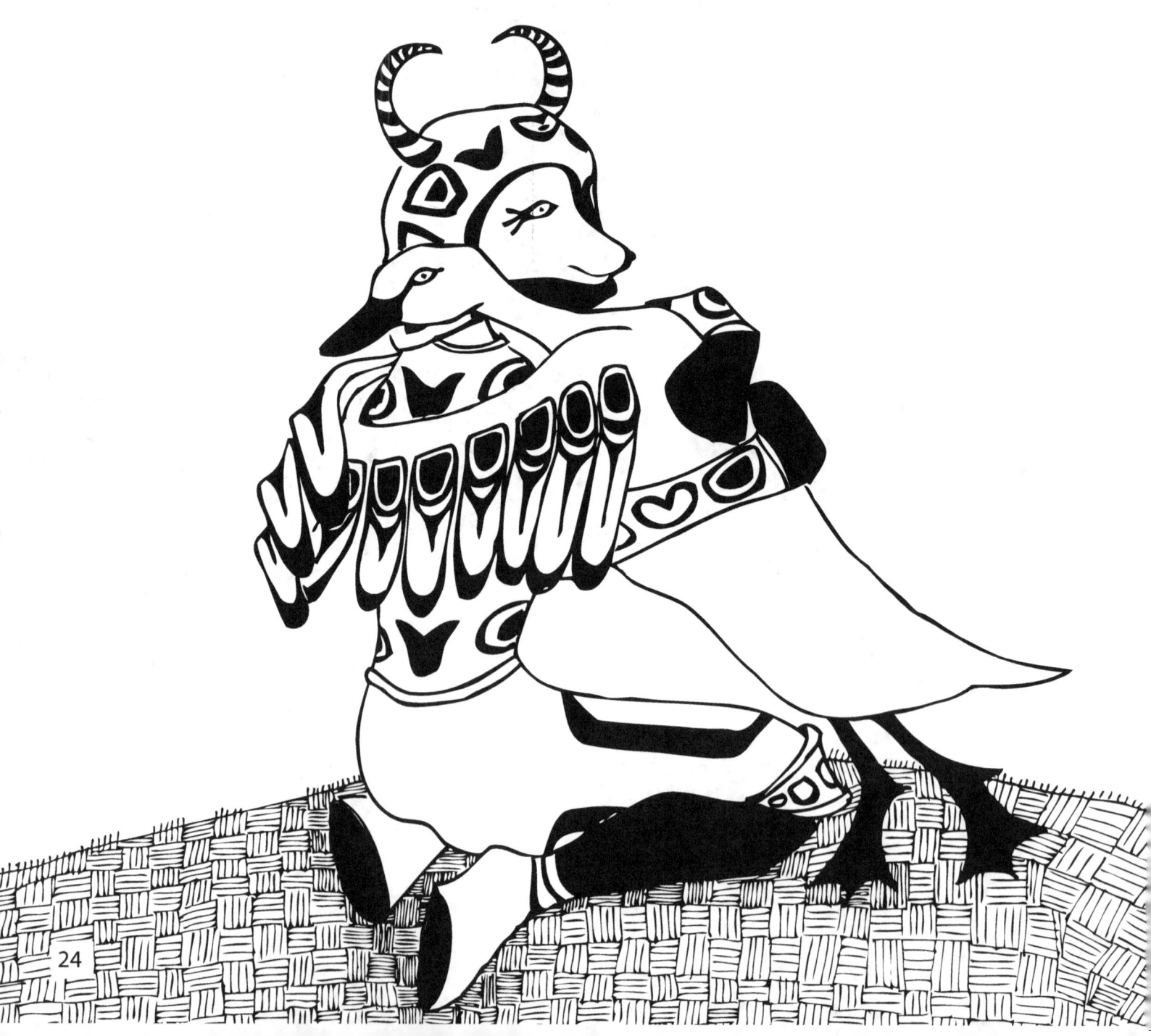

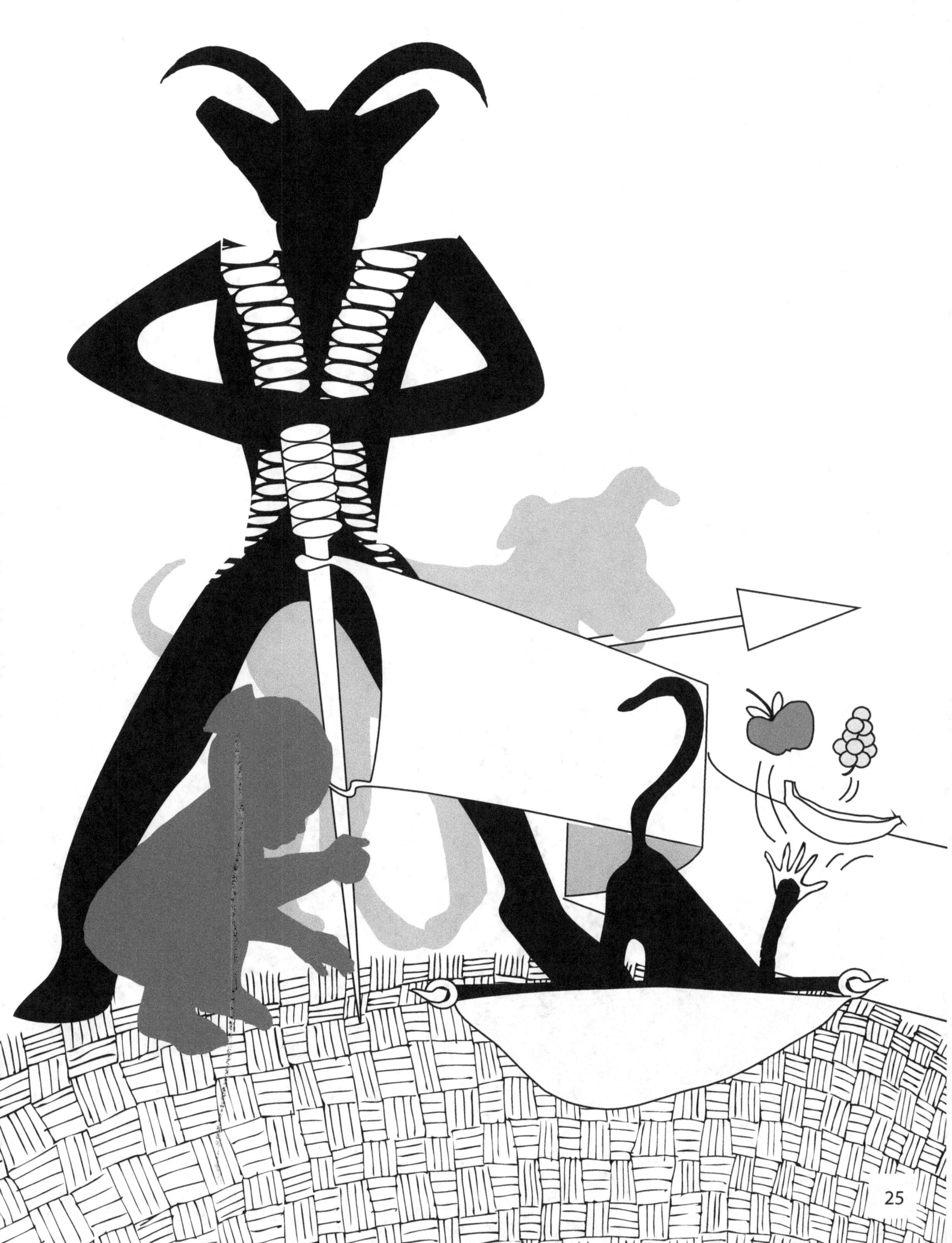

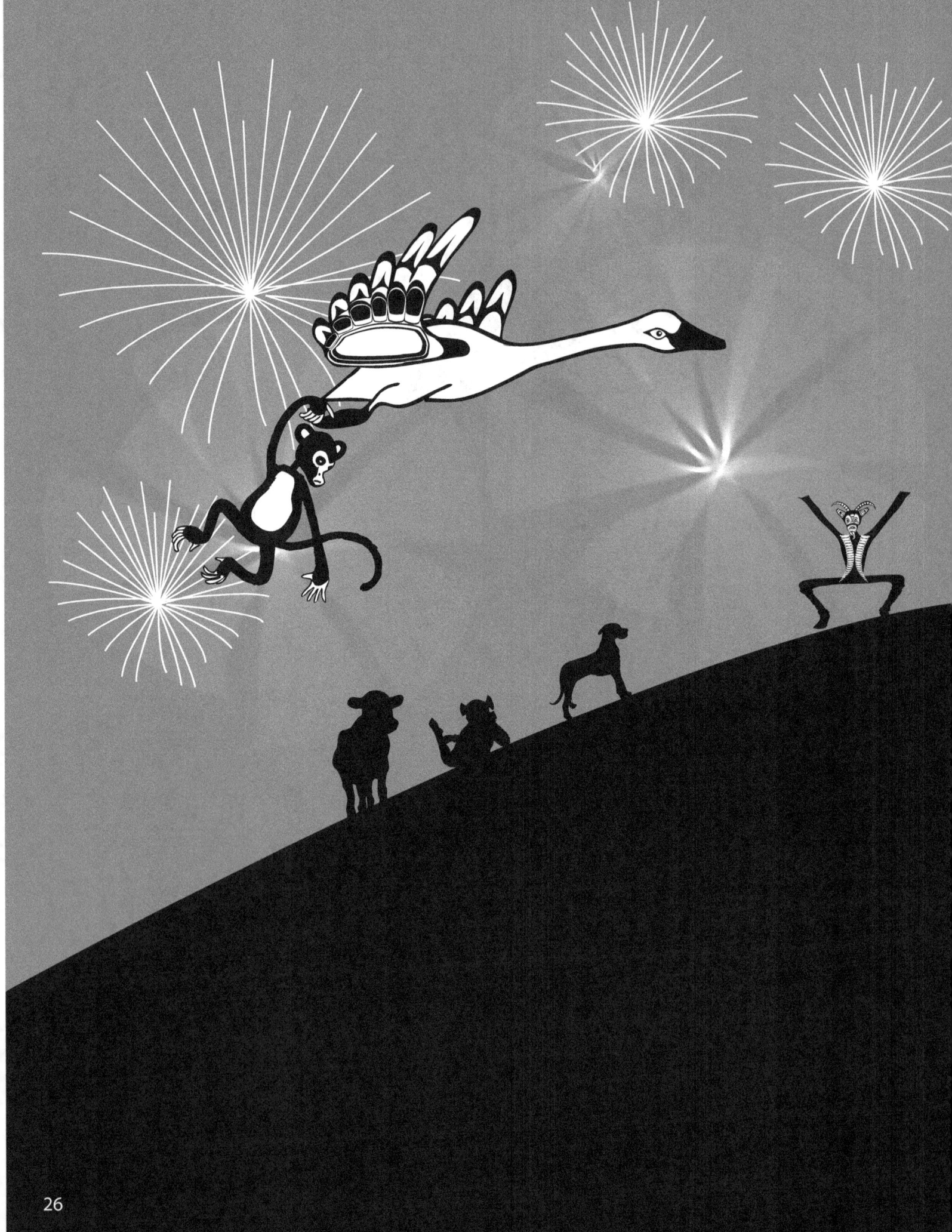

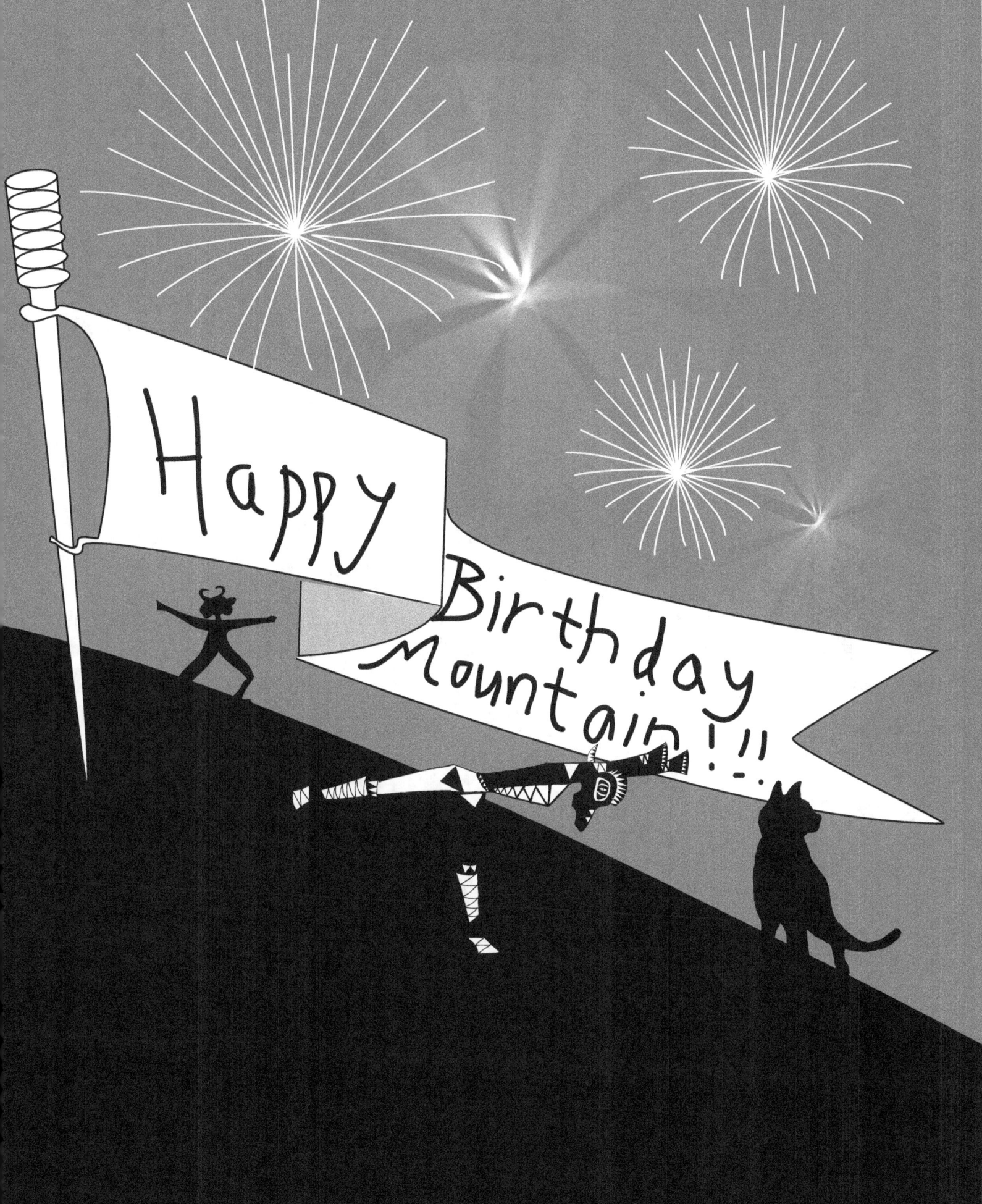

YOGA POSES:

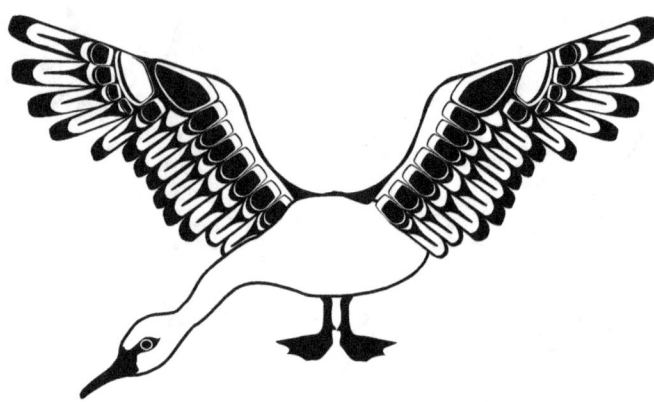

SWAN:

From Mountain pose, take a big breath in, lifting the hands to the sky. On the exhale, swan dive forward, with a flat back, bending from the hips, spread your wings wide.

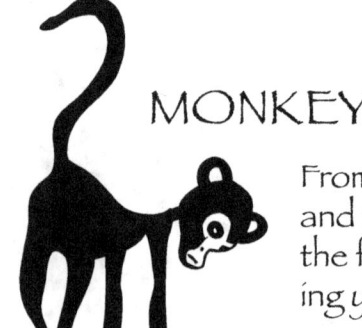

MONKEY POSE:

From Swan, putting the hands on the floor or shins for support, inhale and flatten your back so that it is parallel to the floor. If you can reach the floor, try putting your hands under your feet and inhale, lengthening your back. Try flowing between Mountain, Swan and Monkey.

WARRIOR 1:

From Mountain pose, step back the right foot. The left foot should be pointing straight ahead and the left knee bending toward square. The left knee should not go past the ankle and you should still be able to see your toes. The right foot is behind you at a 45 degree angle. The right leg is straight. Both hips are pointing forward. If this feel like you will fall over, give yourself a little more space so that the feet are not in one line behind each other (that will also help both hips point forward. Raise both arms overhead holding your sword high above you. Do this pose on both sides.

WARRIOR 2:

From Warrior 1, opening the hips and body to face the long edge of your yoga mat. Make sure the legs are still in the same position as in Warrior 1, front leg is bent and the back one is straight. The shoulders are directly above the hips, reach tall through the crown of the head, as the arms reach out over the feet (palms facing down.) The gaze is to the front. Repeat on the other side. Try flowing between Warrior 1 and Warrior 2.

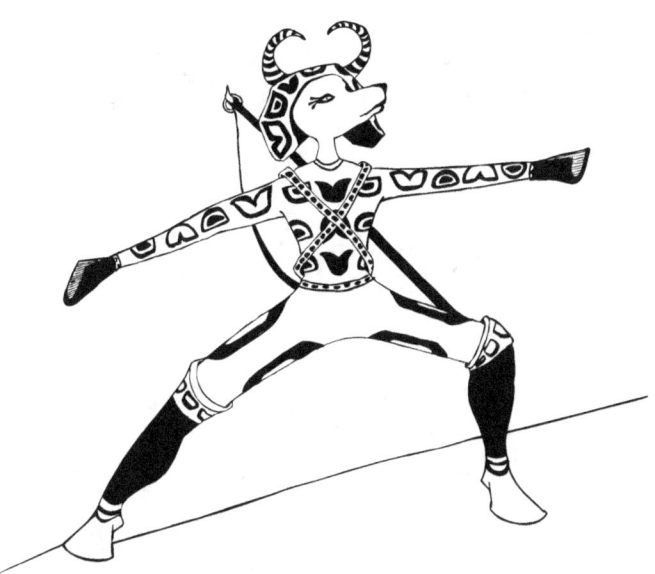

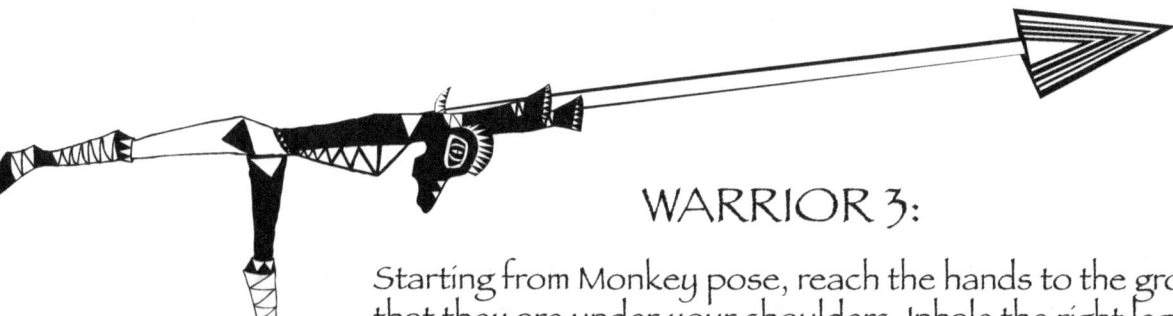

WARRIOR 3:

Starting from Monkey pose, reach the hands to the ground so that they are under your shoulders. Inhale the right leg off the ground. See if you can lift the leg parallel to the ground and still keep both hips pointing to the floor. For an extra challenge, try to lift the hands off the floor bringing them to your sides or even in front of you. Try flowing between Warrior 1 and 3.

GAMES WITH YOGA:

SWAN MIGRATION

Have all the swans in a circle, sitting cross-legged. One child is 'it' and taps each child on the head saying, "monkey" until she finds the swan. The swan must tap the child who is 'it' before the child sits back into the circle where the original swan was sitting.

MONKEYS SAYS

All the children start in a line and one child is "Monkey". The other children must do the pose that Monkey says so long as the phrase "Monkey says" comes before the command. If a player follows a command without "Monkey says," they are put in the forest (where they wait on the side in tree pose for the game to finish.) The last person to stay in the game becomes the new monkey.

WARRIOR TRAINING

Using a pool noodle, have all the warriors in a circle. The warrior holding the sword can decide which warrior they are, then the whole group becomes that warrior. The sword is then passed to the next warrior until everyone who wants a turn has one.

WARRIOR 3 TUNNEL

Pairs of children stand opposite each other, about a body length apart. The partners reach for each other's hands and once they are stable can try to raise a foot and see if they can hold it long enough for a parent or instructor to go through their tunnel.

JEDI TRAINING

For this game you will need as many pool noodles as you have pairs. The pool noodle will be passed between the pairs. The pairs face each other and mirror each other's poses passing the noodle between them.

WARRIOR STOMP

See if your Warriors can stomp to the music by lifting the front heel in your warrior pose. Stomp as you chant "lam" for Warrior 1, "ram" for Warrior 2, and "vam" for Warrior 3. Once the warriors have practiced, split them into groups and have a warrior orchestra, pointing to each group and having them stomp out a beat.
(Note to teachers: The sounds "Lam" "Vam" and "Ram" open the first three chakras. For more chakra fun, try looking for all of the chakra opening sounds on pages 17-21.)

WARRIOR FLOW

The Warriors go through several poses in the book, see if you can find the different poses and link them together as they appear in the book.

GO TO THE TOP OF MOUNTAIN

Quietly resting on the floor, imagine you are on top of mountain with Swan. Swan's full name is Santosha Swan. Santosha means "non judgement" in Sanskrit, the language of yoga. Did your feelings about the warriors change from the beginning of the book to the end of it. Did you think the warriors were friends from the beginning and if not, why not? Imagine you are reading the book again, but this time knowing that the warriors are friends, how does that change the story?

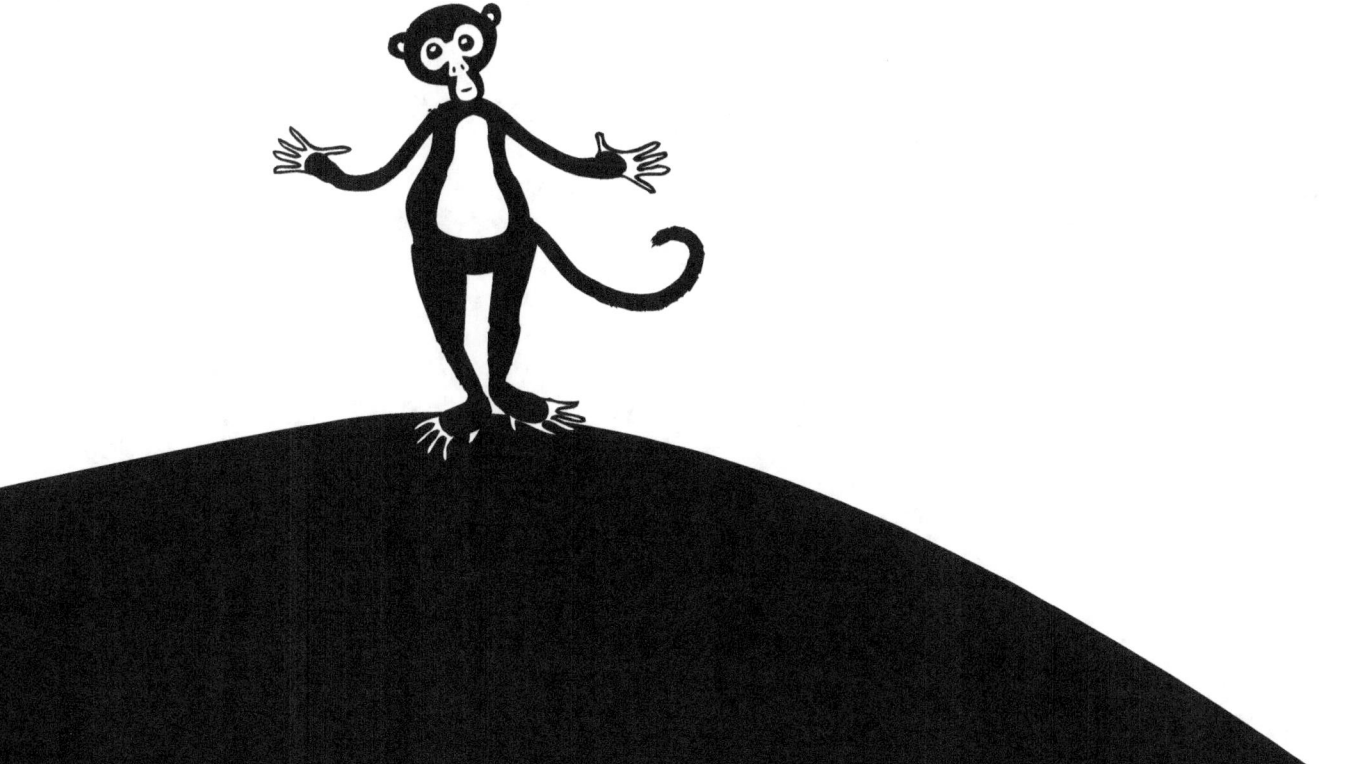

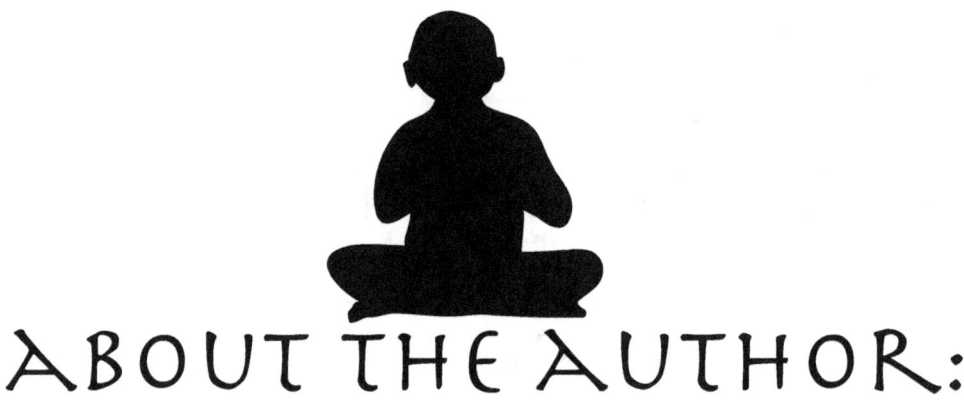

ABOUT THE AUTHOR:

Anna Kekesi-Kim has always loved yoga. She is a certified yoga instructor and homeschooling mother of three boys. She has been a teacher for over twenty years. Anna has always loved the mountains and being outdoors. She also loves to draw and paint. To learn more about her work, visit:

www.annadraws.com

Other titles:
Mountain Moves, a yoga picture book